WAIST MANAGEMENT:

Train Body, Heart, and Mind for Permanent Weight Loss

By Terry L Currier CPT, CH

Disclaimer

The method taught in this Program, *Emotional Freedom Techniques (EFT),* provides impressive results for most people but there is no guarantee it will achieve your goals the way it has for others. Although EFT is a gentle technique, if emotional problems should surface for you while using this program, you should consult your physician and/or therapist regarding your use of EFT.

Copyright
ISBN-13 978-0-9838368-0-3
Published by
TLC Publishing

What They're Saying About *Waist Management* . . .

"Finally, a thoughtful approach to weight management and food cravings that incorporates all the essential components of health and healing, enlisting the mind, body and soul. Whether you want to lose a significant amount of weight or just acquire a healthier lifestyle and eating habits, Waist Management provides the tools and information you need to accomplish your goals. I can't wait to share this holistic resource with my clients."

Paula Koppel, MS, RNC, GNP

"Waist Management is essential reading for anyone who wants to end their struggle with food and weight. By following this program, you'll discover how to lose weight while increasing your energy, improving your health, and developing greater peace of mind."

Stephen Joseph, Psychotherapist,
EFT Practitioner/Trainer

"Many weight loss programs offer little more than platitudes and outdated information. *Waist Management* is a fresh approach that offers every reader an opportunity to experience vitality, well-being, and permanent weight loss. If you've had a hard time losing weight and keeping it off, this is the book you need to read."

Jason Williams
Personal Trainer

"Terry Currier has created a weight loss program that blends solid research-based information with powerful mind/body techniques. This unique combination of healthy eating and exercise, mindfulness, hypnosis and Emotional Freedom Techniques has produced an approach to weight loss that not only produces safe, effective weight loss, but allows the possibility for emotional healing."

Caitlin Williams, M.Ed., LMHC
Psychotherapist, EFT Practitioner/Trainer

"Terry Currier presents a weight loss program that is informative, insightful and effective. By addressing both the physical and emotional factors which prompt overeating, she has created a program that makes successful weight loss possible."

Elena Parsons-Wilson, MS, LMHC
Counselor, Guided Imagery

Dedication

To my dearest daughters,

Sarah and Rebecca

TABLE OF CONTENTS

INTRODUCTION

This weight-loss program is different from any other program you have ever tried. How is it different? It is an approach to weight loss that takes the whole person into account; physically, mentally, emotionally, and spiritually.

So although we will cover nutrition, this is not another diet book. And although we will discuss exercise, this is not another program that promises six-pack abs in eight weeks.

I firmly believe in the importance of eating well and exercising effectively and consistently, and will cover those topics at length. However, losing weight and keeping it off require a major lifestyle change. It is an enormous commitment.

Maintaining this commitment is difficult, if not impossible, unless you can identify and defuse the feelings that send you running to the refrigerator when you are not really hungry. You are likely to repeat the same self-defeating patterns if you don't recognize and change the sabotaging beliefs that keep you stuck in repetitive lose/gain weight cycles. And you may find it difficult to stay motivated if you cannot consistently believe in and imagine yourself achieving your weight-loss goals.

Therefore, in addition to supplying some good, reliable, up-to-date information regarding nutrition and exercise, this program will help you to explore the emotional component of overeating. You will begin to observe the ways you turn to food for comfort, distraction, or reward. You will examine the negative beliefs that continue to cause your weight-loss failures. And you will learn to maintain a positive, healthy image of yourself at your ideal weight, knowing with certainty that you can make that image a reality.

How will you make this happen? In this book I will give you a variety of tools that will engage both your conscious and subconscious mind. Your conscious, reasoning mind will absorb the information offered here. Your willpower, which also belongs to the conscious mind, will fuel your commitment to the process. Finally, through the power of hypnosis you will utilize the incredible power of the subconscious mind to make deep and lasting changes.

While in a wonderfully relaxing trance state, you will receive suggestions that will increase your motivation to eat well and exercise regularly. Guided visualizations will help you develop a healthy, positive image of yourself at your ideal weight. Through hypnosis, you will be able to reduce the stress that can lead to weight gain. And you will also access the wisdom of your deeper mind.

In this book you will also learn how to harness the unbelievable power of the body's energy system. This may be a foreign concept to you, but a blocked or unbalanced energy system can cause tremendous difficulty. With the use of a remarkable technique known as Emotional Freedom Technique, or EFT, you can eliminate food cravings. More importantly, you can use EFT to neutralize painful negative emotions and sabotaging beliefs that stand in the way of lasting weight loss.

Hypnosis and EFT are not magic. You still have to make the lifestyle changes necessary to lose weight. What these techniques do is take the *struggle* out of weight loss. They do this by balancing your energy system, and by aligning the conscious and the subconscious minds so they are in sync. When you stop fighting yourself, weight loss becomes possible.

My Story

For most of my life I suffered from a distorted body image. I always felt I was either overweight or on the verge of becoming fat, and I struggled to keep myself at an unrealistic weight.

Entwined with my distorted self-image was a constant urge to eat. I thought about food all the time, and I spent a lot of mental and emotional energy *not* eating.

In my thirties I met a doctor who insisted I was underweight and urged me to have my body fat percentage tested. Sure enough, my body fat was dangerously low—11.5%. (Minimum BF% for women is 10%.)

I still didn't think I had a problem. After all, how can you be too thin? But the doctor asked me if I knew anything about anorexia, and gave me the name of a dietician she wanted me to see. She really was a good doctor and her concern was sincere, so I made the appointment.

The dietician told me I was not eating enough for my activity level. (I was an aerobic instructor, teaching five or six 90-minute classes per week.) She, too, suggested that I might be anorexic. "What do you mean?" I exclaimed, quite alarmed. "I weigh 112 (at 5' 2"). I don't want to weigh any less."

"Yes," she said, "but what happens when you weigh more?"

That was the big "aha" moment for me, because I knew I freaked out whenever I gained even a pound or two beyond what I considered my ideal weight. (And of course I was always delighted when I weighed less.)

So I began to relax and, much to my doctor's delight, gained five pounds in the next six months.

Nevertheless, I still struggled with food. I still thought about eating a lot of the time. I explored various techniques that might help me let go of this obsession, and discovered hypnosis and EFT. I took up yoga (a natural extension of the meditation practice I was already engaged in). I also began to study nutrition, and discovered that many of my food choices were fueling my food cravings.

I don't really know when it happened, but gradually I lost my preoccupation with food and weight. I stopped obsessing over my next meal as intense food cravings gradually disappeared. And I became comfortable in my body, no longer feeling the need to be rail thin.

This book is the distillation of all that I have learned from my struggles with food and body image. My dearest hope is that you will find it useful, and that it will help you let go of your own struggles so that food can take its place as just one of life's many pleasures.

As you can see, this program is not just about losing weight. It is about healing. It is about restoring your emotional health so that you can become the person you were meant to be. It is about becoming healthy in body, mind, and spirit. It is about feeling as well as looking good. Ultimately, it is about coming home to yourself so that you can know deep peace and lasting happiness.

Onward!

Chapter One
WELCOME TO WAIST MANAGEMENT!

Welcome to Waist Management, a unique program designed by TLC Wellness to train your body, heart, and mind for permanent weight loss. You are about to begin a journey of knowledge, discovery, and healing. You will learn to feed yourself in the way that is healthiest and best suited to you. You will develop an exercise program that is effective and appropriate. You will let go of the old, negative programming that lies at the root of your unhealthy eating habits, and replace it with positive and productive beliefs. And you will heal the wounds that prompt emotional overeating.

Overview

This program is about enhancing physical and emotional health. It involves eating better, moving appropriately, and exploring and healing the emotional problems that have prompted overeating and weight gain.

Each chapter in this manual will cover an aspect of weight loss: nutrition, exercise, mindfulness, stress, resistance, and emotional eating. Below is a brief summary of each of these topics.

Nutrition
The ideal food plan includes lots of vegetables, a moderate amount of fruit and whole grains, and an adequate amount of protein and healthy fat. It also minimizes refined flour, sugar, and processed food.

There is a lot of controversy about the ideal proportions of carbohydrate, protein and fat that should be consumed daily. This author takes the position that fat does not make you fat, but that an abundance of refined carbohydrates do. An excessive amount of flour (even whole wheat), and sugar (of any kind), raises your insulin levels to such a degree that your body will be more likely to store what you eat as fat instead of using it for fuel. These foods can also make you hungrier and increase food cravings.

The amount of food you eat also affects how much fat you store. However, there is a direct correlation between what you eat, how often you are hungry, and what foods you crave. Making healthy food choices will make it easier to eat less.

Integrate the food plan slowly into your life. This is especially imperative if the information provided is new or different. Gradual changes are more likely to be lasting changes.

Exercise
Exercise is an essential component of any healthy, successful weight-loss endeavor, but this does not mean that you have to spend hours in the gym. It does entail identifying activities that you enjoy and then setting up a program that is safe, effective, and realistic for you.

We are all meant to move. Some of us enjoy being physically active more than others. But exercise does not have to be something you trudge through. Walk. Dance. Ride a bike. Then add two, 20 to 30 minute resistance-training sessions per week. The benefits are enormous and the time and effort you put into your fitness program will not only help you lose weight, but will improve your mood, reduce stress, and make you a healthier, happier, and more joyous person.

Start slowly here, too, if you are not currently engaged in a fitness program. Find a way to fit exercise into your life. It really does not have to take up a lot of your time, but does need to become a healthy habit, just like brushing your teeth.

Mindfulness

Losing weight is a matter of eating only when you are physically hungry and then stopping when you have had enough. In order to accomplish this, you must learn to pay attention.

This means that when you feel the urge to eat, you tune into that desire and develop the ability to figure out if it stems from real, physical hunger. If it does, you eat slowly and mindfully so that you can actually taste and enjoy your food, sense fullness, and stop eating when you have had enough.

If the urge to eat is born of a need for comfort, distraction, or some other emotional need, pausing and tuning into your feelings can allow you to address those feelings without turning to food to numb them.

Pay attention to thoughts, feelings, sensations, and to the eating process itself. Engage fully in your experiences. Mindful practices such as meditation and yoga, while not required, can be enormously helpful.

Stress

Stress usually plays a significant role in the impulse to overeat. Examining the effects of stress and developing ways to manage it will not only reduce compulsive eating, but also bring more peace and balance into your life.

Resistance

Resistance will always rear its ugly head sooner or later. If this were not so, weight loss would not be such a long and arduous task for so many. Even the most successful weight-loss journey usually consists of two steps forward and one step back.

The impulse to judge and blame yourself when you slide back into old eating patterns can bring your weight-loss efforts to a complete halt. It is much more helpful and appropriate to see it as a normal part of the weight-loss process. Looking at your resistance, naming it, and learning from it is far more beneficial. Combining this with a healthy dose of self-acceptance and forgiveness will allow you to move forward once again.

Emotional Eating

If you frequently find yourself eating or thinking about eating when you are not hungry, you are probably prompted by emotional issues that you may or may not be aware of. Here is a list of possibilities:

- Uncomfortable feelings arising from your current situation, such as stress, anxiety, grief, frustration, or anger
- Unresolved painful memories from the past
- Innate feelings of shame, guilt, or unworthiness
- A belief that it is unsafe to change your eating habits or to be thinner

To help you deal with these challenging issues, and to assist you in making the lifestyle changes necessary to permanent weight loss, you will learn two very powerful transformational techniques: hypnosis and Emotional Freedom Techniques (EFT).

Hypnosis and Emotional Freedom Techniques (EFT)

Learning about the correct way to eat and keep fit is one thing. Actually applying this knowledge is quite another. Here is where hypnosis and EFT can make a powerful difference in your ability to maintain your weight loss efforts. With regular practice these two methods can make it much easier to change your eating and exercise habits and to make these changes a permanent part of your life. They can also lead to self-discovery and healing.

What is Hypnosis?

Hypnosis is a trance state characterized by extreme suggestibility, relaxation, and heightened imagination. It is most often compared to daydreaming, or the feeling of "losing yourself" in a book or movie. You are fully conscious, but you tune out most of the stimuli around you, focusing instead on what interests you.

In hypnosis we work with both the *conscious* and *subconscious* minds.

The *conscious* mind contains your intellect, your ability to reason, and your capacity for collecting information and analyzing it. It holds your short-term memory. It also includes your willpower, your power of choice, and your commitment to change. This choice, this commitment to work toward your goals, is the first step toward deep and lasting transformation.

The *subconscious* mind holds your imagination, your intuition, and all of your emotions. It also contains your long-term memory; every experience and all of your interpretations of those experiences are stored in the subconscious mind. It also manages the autonomic systems of the body; it controls your digestive system, your cardiovascular system, etc. Whatever happens to you physically that is not within your conscious control is handled by the subconscious.

During hypnosis, the body enters a deeply relaxed state. Once this happens, the wall between the conscious and the subconscious minds becomes more permeable, allowing suggestions to plant themselves deeply and effectively in the subconscious. As a result, profound and lasting changes can take place. You are also able to access the wisdom inherent in your intuition, providing an invaluable source of insight.

Hypnosis feels similar to that lovely state between waking and sleeping. Your breathing slows down as you become more and more relaxed. You might feel lighter or heavier, warmer or cooler. Your extremities may tingle. Sounds tend to fade in and out, and your sense of time may be distorted.

People new to hypnosis are often afraid that it will make them lose control, become unconscious, or do things against their will. The truth is that, under hypnosis, you can never be forced to do anything contrary to your belief system. In hypnosis you will receive suggestions that you only accept statements in accordance with your belief system and for your highest good. You will always be in control because all hypnosis is in effect self-hypnosis, and you must be a willing and active participant.

Old habits, attitudes, and beliefs are deeply etched in the subconscious mind and often sabotage your best efforts to lose weight. By accessing the subconscious mind through hypnosis, you can erase these deep-seated and outdated ways of thinking and replace them with newer, more positive, and ultimately more effective thoughts and beliefs. You can also access the knowledge and insight offered by your intuition It can give you direction and guidance that is not accessible to you during normal conscious awareness.

Hypnosis Recordings

You are strongly urged to practice self-hypnosis everyday by listening to the free hypnosis recording provided with this book. It is entitled "Freedom from Excess Weight." The website page that contains this downloadable recording can be found in the appendix. You will be able to save the recording on your computer, after which you can either burn it to a blank CD or download it onto your mp3 player.

This recording contains motivational messages and suggestions that include:
- Making appropriate lifestyle changes such as eating well and exercising
- Imagining how great you will look and feel at your ideal weight
- Practicing self-care

You can purchase other recordings by using this link to the TLC Weight Loss website: *www.tlcweightloss.net/products.php*. These recordings focus on the various aspects of weight loss presented in Waist Management. For example, "Exercise Motivation," as the name implies, provides motivation to exercise regularly and appropriately. And "Mindful Eating" stresses the importance of paying attention to hunger and fullness signals, and to the eating process itself.

Some of my previous clients have found "Freedom from Excess Weight" quite effective and had no need or desire to use any other hypnosis recordings. Others have found it helpful to listen to a variety of recordings. Everyone is different. Decide what is most useful to you.

Descriptions of these recordings can be found in Appendix C, and at this website address: *www.tlcweightloss.net/products.php*

When to Practice Self-Hypnosis

The best way to incorporate self-hypnosis into your life is to choose a time of day when you can be alone and undisturbed, and practice every day at that time whenever possible. Let this be a practice of deep relaxation, restoration, and self-care.

If time is tight, you can listen to the hypnosis recording of your choice as you go to sleep. Since the subconscious mind is fully engaged while you are sleeping, you will get many of the same benefits that you would if awake. (Because hypnosis is so relaxing, many of my clients use their hypnosis CDs as sleeping aids!)

At the end of the recording you will hear:

"If you are prepared to sleep, you shall sleep deeply and peacefully, and wake up refreshed and well-rested. Otherwise, in a few moments you will come out of trance."

Nevertheless, hypnosis is a more powerful and effective experience if you are awake for it. Besides, it is such a lovely, calming experience that you will find it a great way to begin your day or provide a restful break in your busy schedule.

What is EFT?

In simplest terms, Emotional Freedom Techniques, or EFT, is an emotional form of acupuncture. However, you don't use needles. Instead, you tap with the fingertips to stimulate a series of meridian points, which are the channels of energy, or chi, which runs through the body. While tapping on these points you focus on a specific issue, and on the thoughts, feelings, and/or physical sensations that accompany it. EFT works on the theory that *"the cause of all negative emotions is a disruption in the body's energy system."*

EFT can help you eliminate cravings for those foods which, when eaten in excess, cause weight gain. It can also neutralize the uncomfortable emotions that drive you to overeat. It can negate sabotaging beliefs regarding your ability to lose weight, and resolve the contradictory feelings you may have about becoming thin. And it can help you explore and work through any deeper emotional issues you may harbor that prompt you to use food for comfort or distraction.

Diligent and regular practice of EFT can help you to achieve the following:
- Eliminate food cravings
- Neutralize uncomfortable feelings
- Explore and heal past memories
- Uncover negative, unproductive beliefs and replace them with more positive and effective ones
- Increase self acceptance, forgiveness, and appreciation

EFT will be explained more fully in Chapter Two.

Practice EFT every day. Make it a part of your daily routine. Find at least five to ten minutes a day to make use of the technique. Get in the habit of using it throughout the day.

How This Program Works

Here is an overview of the TLC Waist Management program:
- Educate yourself regarding the healthiest way to eat.
- Decrease consumption of junk food; eat more of healthier alternatives.
- Use EFT and hypnosis daily. These will be extremely helpful in taking the struggle out of the weight-loss process.
- Develop mindfulness regarding (1) emotions that may prompt overeating and (2) the eating process itself.
- When the nutritional foundation has been laid, explore the emotional aspects of overeating. This may require healing events from your past that fuel your present struggles with weight and food. EFT will aid this process.
- Look at beliefs that sabotage your weight-loss efforts. EFT can be tremendously helpful in changing these beliefs.
- Examine the role that stress plays in overeating and develop ways to bring more peace and balance into your life. Practice self-care.
- Incorporate exercise into your life.

Turning Knowledge into Action
As you educate yourself about these issues, you will be given specific instructions about the best way to apply the information. Each chapter ends with a **"Call to Action"** so that you can put into practice what you have learned.

Can This Program Work for Me?
Absolutely! This powerful and easy-to-use program can be very effective. It offers you the tools for addressing the blocks that have previously kept you from success. But, like any other pro-

gram, you will have to use the tools consistently. Consider committing to the following:

- Practice self-hypnosis and EFT *daily*.
- Change or modify your food plan.
- Exercise.
- Practice mindfulness.
- Manage your stress.
- Explore emotional eating issues.

Hypnosis and EFT are not magic bullets! They will not take the effort out of weight loss. However, they will remove the *struggle*. By changing your habits and beliefs on a subconscious level, and by repairing the disruptions in your energy system, you can stop working against yourself and begin to align with your deepest desires, your highest good, and your ideal weight!

Tracking Your Progress
There are several ways to track your progress, and this should be done at least once a month.

- **Weigh yourself regularly.** Once a week works for most. But if you are emotionally distraught by the rise and fall of the scale, once a month will be fine. Just stay aware of and record your progress.
- **Take measurements.** Take these measurements:
  o **Chest** - Standing, measure with breath out, just above the nipple.
  o **Waist** - Standing, measure at the narrowest point or at the midway point between the top of the hip bone and the bottom of the ribcage.
  o **Hips** - Measure at the largest girth, where the buttocks protrude the most.
  o **Thigh** - Standing, measure at the largest girth, just below the buttocks.
- **Measure your Body Fat Percentage**. When you lose weight, your goal should be to *lose fat* and *retain or gain lean muscle mass*. Not only will you look better as you

slim down, but your metabolism will run optimally. You can read more about this in Chapter Eleven.

Measure your body fat in one of these two ways:
- o Find a personal trainer who can take measurements with a skinfold caliper.
- o Purchase a Bioelectrical Impedance (BEI) Analyzer. Some scales, such as the Tanita BF-682 Scale and Body Fat Monitor, will measure body fat as well as weight.

Record these results in the *Waist Management Weight Loss Log*, located on the "**Resources**" page of my website: *www.tlcweightloss.net/resources.php*

CALL TO ACTION

1. See the appendix for directions on downloading the free hypnosis mp3 entitled "Freedom from Excess Weight." Burn it as a CD or transfer it to your mp3 player.

2. Listen to this recording every day.

3. Weigh yourself, take your measurements, and have your body fat percentage measured. Record the results. Continue to monitor your progress by weighing yourself once a week and taking your measurements and body fat percentage once a month.

Chapter Two
EMOTIONAL FREEDOM TECHNIQUES

In this chapter you will learn about Emotional Freedom Techniques, or EFT. This simple yet powerful energy method, developed by Gary Craig, can be an enormously helpful tool for losing weight. You can use it to eliminate food cravings and neutralize uncomfortable feelings that prompt you to overeat. You can also use it to transform self-sabotaging beliefs and heal past wounds that can lead to overeating patterns.

What Is EFT?

In simplest terms, EFT is a psychological form of acupuncture. Like acupuncture, it involves the stimulation of physical meridians. According to traditional Chinese medicine, meridians are channels of energy that run throughout the body and correspond to the body's organs. The life energy that flows through the meridians is called *chi* in Chinese, and the goal of acupuncture is to ensure that the chi flows freely and naturally. However, there are several key differences between acupuncture and EFT.

- Instead of using needles, you tap on or rub certain meridian acupoints on the hands, face, head, and upper body.
- As you do so, you focus on a specific emotional problem or physical ailment and create a statement that describes the issue.
- You administer this technique to yourself. You are an active participant in your healing process.

The core theory of EFT is a belief that all discomfort, whether physical or emotional, is caused by a disruption in the energy system. By tapping on specific acupoints and mentally focusing on the issue at hand, you can dissolve the disruption or blockage, bringing about relief.

Albert Einstein discovered that everything in existence, including our bodies, is composed of energy. If we accept that this energy systematically runs in channels throughout the body, and that the free flow of this energy is paramount to physical and emotional health, then it makes sense that any method that allows the energy to flow freely can bring about tremendous healing.

Every thought or emotion that you experience causes a reaction in a particular area of your brain. Joy or sadness, love or jealousy—all have distinctive counterparts in the way your neurons fire. When you stimulate specific points on your skin by tapping or rubbing, it sends electromechanical signals directly to your brain. If you simultaneously hold in your mind a situation that triggers an unwanted emotional response, you can actually change your brain's response to that situation.

Because our physical bodies and our emotions are connected, repairing an emotional issue energetically will often heal a corresponding physical problem, and visa versa. EFT can be utilized to successfully heal a number of hard-to-treat psychological problems, such as depression, anxiety, phobias, and PTSD (post-traumatic stress disorder). It can also be applied to the elimination of physical pain, and to increasing range of motion in a joint or muscle compromised by injury.

It is also a wonderful tool for reducing the stress of everyday life. It can reduce your anger, ease your frustration, replace anxiety with calmness, and bring tremendous peace into your life.

This model of healing has largely been ignored by Western medicine and psychology. It therefore may seem at odds with your current view of healing and transformation, and you may have doubts about its usefulness. Keep an open mind as you move through the various EFT protocols. It is an unconventional approach, yet it frequently produces visible improvement and often works where other approaches fail. You may be pleasantly surprised that such a nontraditional technique can be so effective.

My own experience with EFT has put me in total awe of its amazing power to change the way I perceive and feel about any situation in which I experience anxiety, anger, guilt, or fear. I have improved my eating habits and greatly improved my relationship with food and with my body. I have healed old wounds and painful memories, allowing me to live my life more in the present moment, instead of seeing my experiences through the prism of the past. In short, it has transformed my life, and continues to do so. And it can do the same for you.

EFT Basics: The EFT Protocol

Overview
Below are the five basic steps you will be following.

1. Identify an issue that is causing you physical or emotional distress.

2. Focus on your issue and assess the intensity of your distress.

3. Craft and then vocalize a statement that accurately describes how you are feeling, adding an affirmation of positive self-regard.

4. Tap on nine specific points while remaining focused on your issue.

5. Reassess the level of distress after a round of tapping, and repeat the tapping sequence if necessary.

Let's examine the details of this procedure.

EFT Step-by-Step

Tune into a specific problem or issue you wish to treat.

Rate the intensity of your distress on a scale of zero to ten. This scale is known as *SUD,* or Subjective Units of Distress.

Tap the **Karate Chop Point (KC)** of either hand 10 to 15 times while saying *"Even though I have this problem, I deeply and completely accept myself."* Repeat this two more times. This is called the *Set-Up*:

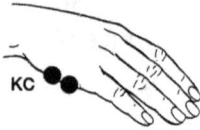

Tap each of the following points 10 to 15 times, while repeating the **Reminder Phrase,** *"this problem"*: *Eyebrow (EB), Side of Eye (SE), Under Eye (UE), Under Nose (UN), Chin (CH), Collarbone (CB), Underarm (UA),* and *Top of Head (H).* See the next page for a more detailed description of these points.

EYEBROW (EB)	
SIDE OF EYE (SE)	
UNDER EYE (UE)	
UNDER NOSE (UN)	
CHIN (CH)	
COLLARBONE (CB)	
UNDERARM (UA)	
HEAD (H)	

Take a deep breath. Rate the SUD level again. If your SUD level is zero to two, you may stop. If it is two or higher, repeat the revised Set-Up Phrase, "Even though I still have some of this problem, I deeply and completely accept myself."

Tap all the points again, repeating the revised Reminder Phrase, "This remaining problem."

Reassess the SUD level and repeat if necessary.

EFT POINTS

Karate Chop Point (KC): In the middle of the fleshy part on the outside of the hand, between the top of the wrist bone and the base of the baby finger

Eyebrow (EB): At the beginning of the eyebrow, just above and to one side of the nose

Side of Eye (SE): On the bone bordering the outside corner of the eye

Under Eye (UE): On the bone under the eye, about an inch below the pupil

Under Nose (UN): On the small area between the bottom of the nose and the top of the upper lip

Chin (CH): Midway between the point of the chin and the lower lip

Collarbone: The junction between the sternum (breastbone), collarbone, and first rib. Place your forefinger on the U-shaped notch at the top of the breastbone. Move down toward the naval about an inch and then go to the right or left one inch.

Underarm (UA): On the side of the body, at a point even with the nipple (for men), or in the middle of the bra strap (for women)

Top of Head (H): On the top and center of the head. Tap in a circular motion around the crown of the head.

Using EFT to Eliminate Food Cravings

Now that you have a general idea of how the method works, let's use it to let go of your desire for those unhealthy foods that are sabotaging your weight-loss efforts.

Choose a food that you often crave; one you know is unhealthy and would like to avoid. It could be candy, chips, ice cream, or any junk food you frequently struggle with. Now look at it, smell it, imagine eating it. Using the SUD rating, assess the intensity of your craving.

1. The Set-Up: Tap 10 to 15 times on the Karate Chop point while repeating the Set-Up Phrase:

> *"Even though I really want this _____, I deeply and completely accept myself."*

Or you might say

> *"Even though I have this strong craving for _____, I deeply and completely accept myself."*

The words you choose need to be the ones that best reflect how you feel about your desire for the particular food at this time. Do this three times.

2. The Sequence: With two or three fingers, lightly tap about 10 to 15 times on the points indicated in the diagram. As you tap each point, use the Reminder Phrase, which is an abbreviated version of the Set-Up Phrase. It will help focus on the craving.

"I really want this _____"

   Or

"This craving for_____"

(It doesn't matter which hand you use or which side of the body you tap on.)

3. Breathing, Observing, Reassessing: Stop, pause, and take a deep breath. Now check out the craving. Has the smell changed? Has the intensity of the craving decreased? If so, what number would you now give it on a scale of zero to ten?

Let's assume that the craving has decreased, but not gone away. For example, your number may have started at nine and decreased to four. You will continue the process as follows.

4. Subsequent Rounds: Do another round of tapping, changing the Set-Up Phrase to acknowledge that some of the craving is gone, but some remains. While tapping on the Karate Chop Point, say the Set-Up Phrase as follows:

"Even though I still want _____, I deeply and completely accept myself."

   Or

"Even though I still have some craving left for _____, I deeply and completely accept myself."

And then change the Reminder Phrase to

"Still want this _____"

Or

"This remaining craving for _____"

Keep tapping until you have brought the craving down to a two
or lower. And that's it.

When to Tap and for How Long

Set aside about ten minutes a day to tap on your food issues.
Morning works best for most people, but choose whatever time
of day works best for you. The important principle is consistency.
Start by focusing on and eliminating cravings for the foods you
struggle with the most. If you don't have the specific food you
want to tap on in front of you, then imagine it; see it, smell it, and
taste it in your mind's eye. Tap the craving down to a two, or as
low as possible during that session.

Assess the level of craving for that particular food the following
day. Note the intensity of the craving. Tap for the food again if
the craving is three or higher. If your craving is gone, choose another food you often struggle with and repeat the tapping proto-
col for cravings. Continue this process until you can successfully
walk away from whatever food you have been trying to resist.
Meanwhile, you will also be adding healthier foods to your diet, as
explained in Chapter Three.

As you move through this practice, note any resistance or feelings
of deprivation or resentment that show up. Just pay attention to
any thoughts or feelings that arise. Be curious. Later on in this
program you will learn to explore and work with these issues using EFT. For now, just notice them.

A journal can be very helpful at this point. Observe and record your feelings, without judgment or expectations. Your journal can provide you with useful information. Later on, you can use EFT to clear away feelings that surfaced as you wrote in your journal.

Tapping for Cravings in the Moment
Food temptations often show up unexpectedly, and tapping can be a great tool for combating the urge to eat inappropriately. If there are other people around, you can learn to tap surreptitiously. See the section below on "Covert EFT."

<u>Using EFT to Eat Less</u>

EFT for "Dangerous" Times
The next way I suggest you use EFT is to prepare yourself for the times of day when you feel the most vulnerable to overeating.

Is late-night snacking your problem? Try using statements such as the following:

"Even though I love to snack on _____ at night, I deeply and completely accept myself."

"Even though I love to relax with a bag of _____..."

"Even though I deserve to eat _____ after a hard day..."

"Even though I don't want to give up my late-night snacks..."

"Even though I don't think I can stop eating at night..."

Remember, use words that best reflect *your* thoughts and feelings.

You can use this same method to negate your habit of overeating when you go to a restaurant, a holiday dinner, or on any other occasion that is associated with overindulging.

Here are some more statements you might find useful:

"Even though I want to eat whatever is in front of me, I deeply and completely accept myself."

"Even though I want to eat like a pig when I go out to dinner . . ."

"Even though it's hard to stick to my diet around other people . . ."

"Even though I always eat too much when I go to my mother's house, and it makes her happy when I eat a lot . . ."

Again, don't worry about getting the words just right. Use phrases that reflect how you feel about your food struggles.

EFT Aimed at General Dysfunctional Eating Patterns

Another helpful EFT practice is to create one or two statements that reflect your key struggles with food. Although it is usually important to be as specific as possible when using EFT, global EFT statements used daily in the early weeks can be very helpful for changing your eating patterns.

"Even though I think about food all the time . . ."

"Even though I am totally obsessed with food . . ."

"Even though I can't control how much I eat . . ."

"Even though I always eat a lot and won't practice portion control . . ."

"Even though the only time I'm happy is when I'm eating . . ."

"Even though I'd rather eat than do anything else..."

"Even though food is my friend..."

"Even though I eat whenever I'm bored, angry, lonely, etc..."

"Even though I can't stop eating once I start..."

"Even though I always want seconds..."

"Even though I continually pick at food..."

"Even though I want to eat every time I see food..."

Additional Times to Tap

In addition to your focused tapping sessions, it is useful to tap for brief periods throughout the day. Take a few minutes to perform several rounds of tapping, using either the global EFT statements mentioned previously, or the phrases you are using to prepare yourself for those "dangerous times" when you tend to overeat. This will promote a continuous reduction of the emotional blocks that have been creating your eating difficulties.

You may wish to tap during the following times:

- When you get up
- In the shower
- When you use the bathroom
- Before a meal
- At a stoplight
- Before you get out of your car
- Before you fall asleep

General EFT Tips and Suggestions

Covert EFT

Quite often you will need to use EFT when you are in public situations. While I look forward to the day when EFT becomes an everyday tool that everyone can use freely and unselfconsciously, that day may be a ways off. Therefore, below is a list of ways you can tap without looking conspicuous.

- Press, rub, and hold the points instead of tapping.
- Separate your index and middle fingers and rub around your eyes with both hands; the index fingers rubbing the Side of Eye (SE) points, the middle fingers rubbing the Beginning of Eyebrow (BE) points and then continuing Under the Eye (UE). Rub, hold, and breathe.
- Make a fist. Bring the knuckle of your index finger to the Under Nose (UN) point and the knuckle of your thumb to your Chin (CH) point. Rub, hold, and breathe.
- Bring one hand to the upper chest and press both Collarbone points with a thumb and forefinger. By bringing your hand under your arm instead of holding your elbow, you can get the Underarm (UA) point as well. Rub, hold, and breathe.
- You can cross your arms and, while your arms are crossed, reach for the Underarm points. Rub, hold, and breathe.
- Top of Head? Scratching or massaging your head won't look strange.
- Although we don't usually use these points in the general EFT procedure (unless you're using Gary Craig's original, longer EFT "Recipe"), there are acupoints on the side of each finger facing the thumb, next the fingernail. You can use your thumb to tap or rub these points unobtrusively.
- For the Karate Chop point, you can fold your hands across your abdomen, one hand over the other, and gently tap or rub with the fingers of the top hand on the Karate Chop point of the other hand.

- Once you are familiar and comfortable with the method, you will be able to mentally tap on each point while saying the appropriate statements silently to yourself. Amazingly enough, you will get the same results as you would if you were physically tapping on each point.

Tapping on the Negative

Quite often people are surprised and a bit concerned about using negative statements. Shouldn't we be focused on the positive?

For EFT to work, you must be tuned into your problem. It's like accessing information from your computer; you need to call up the appropriate "program." This focus allows you to take precise aim at your issue, and is the most effective way to apply EFT.

There is a variation of EFT called the Choices Method, created by Dr. Patricia Carrington. This technique introduces positive affirmations into the EFT process, and will be explained in Chapter Eight. For now, as you learn the method, it is best to practice by simply stating the problem you wish to address.

Self-Acceptance

Saying the self-acceptance phrase feels strange or uncomfortable for some people. However, it is an important part of the EFT method. In the process of developing EFT, it was discovered that when you tap on the Karate Chop point while repeating a self-acceptance statement, the body is more able to process the effects of the tapping. You also don't have to believe in EFT in order for it to work. I will expand on the topic of self–acceptance in Chapter Eight.

The EFT Manual

You will find it tremendously helpful to purchase Gary Craig's "The EFT Manual." It is a marvelous introduction to this extremely powerful technique. Although EFT is a very simple and user-friendly method, there is an art to it, which you can learn by reading Gary's book and by practicing EFT daily. (There are more wonderful books on EFT listed in the Resource section of this book.)

CALL TO ACTION

1. Begin using EFT daily.
   - For food cravings, choose one food each day and tap the food craving down to two or lower. Check for any remaining cravings for that food the next day. If there are none, go onto another food.
   - Tap for "dangerous times," preparing yourself for the times of day and situations when you are most vulnerable to overeating.
   - Choose one or more of the general overeating themes that seem true for you, and tap on those.

Set aside about ten minutes each morning for these tapping themes. Then tap several times throughout the day, as described above.

2. Continue to listen daily to the hypnosis recording, "Freedom from Excess Weight."

Chapter Three
THE FOOD LISTS

A balanced, moderate intake of calories is the best prescription for healthy weight loss. An optimal, balanced diet includes:

- an adequate amount of healthy protein and fat.
- a minimal amount of sugar or refined grains.
- lots of vegetables.
- some fruit and nuts.
- a small amount of starchy carbohydrates (such as sweet potatoes or oatmeal).

It is important to minimize the quantity of processed foods you consume, opting for foods that are as close to their natural state as possible. Processed foods are full of the refined grains, sugars, and unhealthy fats you want to avoid.

For some, weight loss will progress quite nicely when most refined carbohydrates and unhealthy fats are removed from the diet, and more fruits and vegetables, lean protein, and healthy fat are added. So the next step in the process is to do exactly that.

Below are two lists of foods. The **"Optimal Choices"** list consists of wholesome, nutritious foods that can move you towards healthy weight loss. Begin adding or increasing these in your food plan. On the **"Least Desirable"** list are the foods that have probably contributed to your weight gain in the past. Remove one or two of these per week. Use EFT to eliminate cravings for any of the foods that are difficult to let go of.

Please remember that healthy eating is about *adding* selected foods to your diet, and not just taking foods out. For those of you who have been in low-fat mode, there is a good chance that you are not consuming enough protein and healthy fat, and you will need to add more selections from those food groups. At first, you may find this shift challenging. Rest assured that you will eventually find this manner of eating much more satisfying. Your cravings and your hunger will decrease when you reduce or eliminate the "white stuff"—white flour, rice, pasta, and sugar in all its various forms—and add healthy sources of lean protein and fat.

If you observe feelings of anxiety or deprivation as you read over this list, just note them for now. In the following chapters you will learn to use EFT to neutralize those feelings. You will not have to grit your teeth and rely solely on willpower.

Before we go any further, though, a word about calories. Sometimes veteran dieters get panicky when they are not told exactly how much food they can eat. Relax. In Chapter Five I will get specific about the amount of food you can consume for steady weight loss. For now, focus on eating more of the good stuff and eating fewer foods that cause food cravings and weight gain.

Optimal Choices

Vegetables. These are the best foods to add to your diet. Think in terms of color, and eat lots of colorful foods—red, orange, yellow, and especially green. Vegetables provide fiber, nutrients, antioxidants, phytochemicals, and enzymes. Fresh-squeezed vegetable juice is also a great way to ingest more of these nutritionally dense foods.

The following is a partial list of vegetables to choose from:

alfalfa sprouts, beets, broccoli, Brussels sprouts, cabbage, carrots, cauliflower, celery, collard greens, cucumbers, eggplant, kale, leeks, mushrooms, okra, onions, parsnips, peas, peppers (green/red/yellow), snow peas, spinach, tomatoes

Fruit. Aim for two to three servings of fruit a day. *Apples, apricots, grapefruit, pears,* and *plums* are good choices. *Blueberries, raspberries,* and *strawberries* are also good. However, fruits should not be treated as an "unlimited" item because many of them are high in sugar. Eating too much of them can cause weight gain. Dried fruits are especially high in sugar.

Whole Grains. We eat certain grains, like rice and oatmeal, in their natural state. Others, like wheat, are the main ingredient in breads, pastas, and some cereals. Although you need to watch the size and number of grain servings, they are a rich source of vitamins, minerals, and fiber.

Some of the most wholesome grains are:

barley, brown and wild rice, bulgur, millet, oatmeal, quinoa, whole wheat berries

Seafood. If you can eat seafood several times a week, that's great. Not only is seafood a nutrient-packed source of protein, it's one of the richest sources of omega-3 fatty acids, the super-healthy polyunsaturated fat linked to the reduction of heart disease, depression, and stroke.

However, many people are concerned about the amount of mercury in fish, and rightly so. Mercury is a potent neurotoxin, meaning it can affect all brain functions, including thinking, learning, memory, and mood. The risk factors depend upon the amount of mercury ingested and your ability to get rid of it.

The higher the fish is on the food chain, the higher its mercury content. Consequently, the safest kind of fish to eat is *farmed trout, wild salmon, summer flounder,* and *blue crab.* The most dangerous are shark, swordfish, king mackerel, tilefish, and tuna.

Eggs. Eggs are one of the most nutritious foods money can buy.

They're packed with a range of nutrients, including protein, essential vitamins A, D, E, and the B group, as well as the minerals iron, phosphorus and zinc. Eggs have gotten a bad reputation over the last decade, but a very unfair one. Contrary to popular belief, *dietary cholesterol does not raise serum cholesterol.* So eat and enjoy them; have a couple a day if you'd like. This includes the yolks, which are a tremendous source of nutrients, including phosphatidylcholine. Phosphatidylcholine is needed to form lecithin, which actually helps prevent cholesterol from being oxidized, and is also a superb nutrient for liver health and brain function.

Whey protein powder. Whey protein is a high-quality protein powder made from cow's milk, and is an excellent source of protein. Shakes made with whey protein are a great way to get protein when you are crunched for time and can't prepare a full meal. It is inexpensive and can be added to various foods to increase protein content. People who are have allergies or sensitivities to cow's milk, however, should avoid whey.

Meat and poultry. There are many sources of meat that are easy to incorporate into any meal. Look for lean cuts of *beef, lamb, pork, veal, chicken, turkey,* and *duck.*

There is a growing interest in choosing meat that is healthy and humanely raised, i.e., grass-fed, free range, with no antibiotics. For these products, shop at stores that carry organically raised meats and read labels.

Nuts. Nuts can be a great source of protein, essential fatty acids, and minerals. Be careful though; nuts are high in fat and therefore calorically dense. If possible, avoid salted nuts, since they are easy to overeat and high in sodium. Nevertheless, don't be afraid to garnish a salad with a small handful of walnuts or to spread a tablespoon of cashew butter on your morning toast. *Pecans, almonds,* and *walnuts* have the best mixture of good fats and minerals. Raw *Brazil nuts, cashews, filberts (hazelnuts),* and *macadamia nuts* are also an excellent choice.

Healthy fat sources. Many people who have been following the low-fat diet dogma are woefully under-consuming good fats. Paradoxically, some fats, like the omega-3 fats found in fish and flaxseed, can actually help you *lose* body fat. These fatty acids "sit" on the cell membrane, encouraging other fats to get into the cell where they can be burned for fuel. Below is a partial list of healthy fats and foods that contain healthy fats:

> *avocado, butter, canola oil* (cold or expeller-pressed), *coconut, coconut oil, flaxseed meal, flaxseed oil* (but don't cook with it), *nuts, nut butters, olive oil* (cold pressed, extra-virgin), *seeds, sesame tahini,* and fats found in cold-water fish like *mackerel, salmon, sardines,* and *tuna*

Water. Involved in every cellular process, water is the best weight-loss drink in the world. I recommend drinking about eight glasses a day, with an additional eight ounces for every 25 pounds you are overweight. Keep in mind, though, that you will need to drink more when it's hot out. And when you exercise, you definitely need to drink more—12 to 16 additional ounces.

If you currently drink an inadequate amount of water, begin by adding one or two additional glasses a day and increase slowly over time.

Least Desirable Choices

Anything made with white flour and sugar. This includes most commercial breads, bagels, pastas, muffins, cakes, cookies, candies, snack foods, and soda. It also includes most cereals, with the exception of whole grain sources such as *slow-cooking oatmeal* (also called Old Fashioned), *buckwheat groats (kasha),* and *whole-grain grits.*

Sugar and white flour are low in nutrition and fiber. They are also high-glycemic foods, which means they provoke sharp rises in blood sugar and insulin. Thus they can trigger hunger and food cravings, increasing the likelihood that you will overeat. High-glycemic foods also boost your body's capacity to store food as fat rather than burning it for energy.

A note about whole-wheat products: Once a grain has been pulverized into flour, it becomes a high-glycemic food. So although whole-wheat foods (such as bread and pasta) have more nutrition than their bleached counterparts, they can produce the same consequences as other high-glycemic foods.

A great alternative to bread made with whole-wheat flour is *sprouted wheat bread*. It is produced by sprouting wheat berries and then grinding them into dough. This creates a product higher in protein and fiber, with a lower impact on blood-sugar levels than most other breads. (A good, organic, sprouted-wheat bread is *Ezekiel*.)

Beware of **sugar**, and avoid it as much as possible. Although a few sugars such as honey and molasses have some nutritional and even medicinal value, for all of the reasons stated above, minimize their consumption while you are trying to lose weight.

The amount of sugar in processed foods is often misleading, so read food labels carefully. Below is a list of some of the possible names that may appear on a label. Hint: the words "syrup," "sweetener," and anything ending in *ose* can usually be assumed to be "sugar."

> *barley malt, beet sugar, brown rice syrup, brown sugar, cane juice, confectioners' powdered sugar, corn sweetener, corn syrup, date sugar, dextrin, dextrose, fructose, fruit juice*, galactose, high-fructose corn syrup, honey, invert sugar, lactose, malted barley, mali-tol, maltose, mannitol, maple sugar, microcrystalline, molasses, oli-*

gosaccharides, polydextrose, raisin juice, raw sugar, sorbitol, su-canant, sugarine, turbinado sugar, unrefined sugar, white sugar

If you are looking for a sugar substitute, *Stevia* is a safe, wholesome product, made from the small, green *stevia rebaudiana* plant, an herb found in South America. It has a negligible effect on blood sugar, which is why it is useful for people trying to reduce their sugar intake. Consider trying Stevia if you want a sweetener, however, be aware that not everyone likes the taste.

Fruit juice. Although fruit itself is healthy, once the pulp and fiber have been squeezed out of it, juice itself is not a great choice. It can cause blood sugar and insulin levels to rise dramatically, just as if you had consumed soda. Note that the juices chosen as sweeteners, such as white grape, apple, and pear juices, are among the least nutritious of the juices. By the time they are "concentrated," very little remains except the sugar.

Refined vegetable oils. These are among the worst items on the list. Don't eat or cook with them. The common vegetable oils you find in the supermarket are loaded with toxins and have been falsely marketed as healthy. Avoid refined corn oil, sunflower oil, safflower oil, and soy oil. These fats have been processed to such a degree that they are no longer healthy food choices.

Margarine. Margarine, sometimes referred to as oleo, is a highly refined, hydrogenated product, usually made with vegetable oils. At one time, it was considered healthier than eating butter. Current research shows, however, that it is a trans fat, making it extremely unhealthy. Trans fats raise your "bad" (LDL) cholesterol and lower your "good" (HDL) cholesterol. Manufacturers and restaurants are now responding to pressure to stop using hydrogenated oils. Butter is a better choice.

Of Questionable Value

Dairy

You may have noticed that I have not mentioned dairy products. That is because they are beneficial for some people, but not for others. Although some people tolerate dairy well, an estimated 70% of the world's population is lactose-intolerant. The promotion of milk as a healthy food has more to do with the political power of the dairy industry than it does with the actual nutritional value of dairy products.

Some people who don't tolerate milk and cheese well have no problems with yogurt. However, don't make the mistake of assuming that fruit-flavored yogurt is a good idea. "Fruit" in this context is another word for sugar. Eat plain yogurt, add real fruit, and sweeten with Stevia if you want additional sweetness.

When I mention my reservations about milk, the question I most often hear is, "How will I get my calcium?"

According to Dr. Walter Willet, one of the lead authors of the rigorous Nurses' Health Study, there is no calcium emergency. There's little evidence that getting high amounts of calcium prevents broken bones in the senior population. Consuming 550 ml daily appears to be adequate, and consuming too much can possibly increase the risk of prostrate and ovarian cancers.

It's easy to get your required daily amount from these foods:

Calcium in Beans
- Tofu 150g: 350 ml
- Cooked soybeans 1 cup: 130 ml
- White beans 3/4 cup: 120 ml
- Navy beans ¾ cup: 94 ml
- Black turtle beans 3/4 cup: 75 ml
- Chickpeas (*chole, garbanzos*) 3/4 cup: 58 ml

Calcium in Nuts
- Almonds, roasted 1/4 cup: 93 ml
- Almond butter 2 Tbsp: 88 ml
- Sesame seeds 1/4 cup: 50 ml

Calcium in Vegetables and Fruits
- Cabbage/bok choy 1/2 cup: 190ml
- Turnip greens 1/2 cup: 104 ml
- Broccoli 1/2 cup: 33 ml
- Okra 1/2 cup: 65 ml
- Oranges 1/2 cup: 52 ml

Alcohol. Although there are well-documented benefits from moderate alcohol consumption, you may want to take it out of your diet while you're trying to lose weight, for two reasons: you will be better off without the extra calories, and you might find yourself eating more because of the way alcohol can lower your inhibitions.

CALL TO ACTION

1. Continue to reduce your cravings for junk food with EFT, including those found in the "Least Desirable Choices" list. Begin to introduce/increase food selections from the "Optimal Choices" list. Remember, this is not just about taking food out of your diet, but adding healthy ones in. You will notice that as you add more protein, vegetables, and healthy fats, your cravings for refined carbohydrates will decrease.

2. Continue to practice EFT as directed, for times when you're likely to overeat or consume unhealthy foods. Also, use your general overeating statements when you practice EFT.

3. Continue to listen daily to the hypnosis recording, "Freedom from Excess Weight." or to the recording of your choice. (See Appendix. You may find the hypnosis recording of "Eat, Drink, and Be Healthy" especially helpful.)

Chapter Four
NUTRITION BASICS

In this chapter we will cover the basics of good nutrition. These include a description of the major food groups: what they are (fat, protein, carbohydrates, and water), how they function in the body, and which foods they are found in. It will also explain what a well-balanced diet looks like and suggest the percentages from each food group you would consume for optimal health and weight loss.

There is considerable controversy about how much to eat from each food group. Previous dietary guidelines from the USDA to eat a low-fat, high-grain diet have been challenged by many doctors and nutritionists, who now recommend a diet higher in protein and lower in grains. This is a very important topic as it relates to weight loss. I will discuss the different sides of the issue and make my own recommendations.

One Size Does Not Fit All

Let me be clear; there is no one perfect diet for everyone. A one-size-fits-all approach to weight loss is not suitable or effective. We are all unique individuals. There are many factors that influence our ability to lose weight. These include metabolism, activity level, heredity, age, gender, hormonal responses, neurochemistry, and food sensitivities.

Nevertheless, I will present guidelines for healthy eating that work well for most people. Use these guidelines by experimenting and adjusting them to create an eating plan that works for your body.

Consider Both Quality and Quantity

Some nutritionists claim that if you eat certain types of food and avoid others, you will automatically lose weight. Others insist that a calorie is a calorie, and that it doesn't matter what type of food you eat as long as you eat less than you previously have.

You need to consider both quality and quantity. If you ingest more calories than you burn, you will gain weight, and if you eat fewer, you will lose. But the type of food you eat is also significant. What you eat affects your food cravings, sense of hunger and satiety, fat storage, self-control, mood, and overall health.

Nutrition 101

Food is divided into two major categories; macronutrients and micronutrients. The macronutrients are as follows:
- Carbohydrates: fruits, vegetables, legumes, milk, all grains (bread, pasta, rice, etc.), and all forms of sugar
- Protein: meat, poultry, fish, cheese, nuts, legumes, milk, cheese, whey powder, and soy products
- Fat: butter, oil, nuts, and animal fat
- Water

You will notice some duplication in these lists. Legumes contain both carbohydrates and protein. Nuts are primarily a fat, but include protein. Dairy products are a combination of all four macronutrients.

Micronutrients are the vitamins and minerals found in most foods that are required in microgram quantities in order for the human body to function correctly. Vitamin A, for instance, helps you see well. Vitamin K aids normal blood clotting. There are a total of 28 micronutrients.

Some micronutrients are closely involved in specific body functions related to weight management. For example, Vitamins B1, B5, and B6 aid in metabolism, while chromium improves insulin sensitivity. Selenium and iodine contribute to thyroid hormone function. Metabolic efficiency, insulin response, and thyroid function can all influence weight and appetite.

The emphasis in this book will be on macronutrients. For more information on the micronutrients that impact weight loss, I refer you to Jonny Bowden's chapter on supplements in his highly informative book, *Shape Up! The Eight-Week Program To Transform Your Body, Your Health and Your Life.*

Carbohydrates

Carbohydrates, or saccharides, are sugars and starches. During digestion, carbohydrates break down into glucose, which is the body's primary source of fuel. (When you restrict the number of carbohydrates you eat, however, the body will make glucose from protein.) Carbohydrates are found primarily in plant foods, such as fruits, vegetables, legumes, grains, and all forms of sugar. They also exist in milk and milk products.

Fruits and vegetables also contain the majority of the vitamins, minerals, phytochemicals, and antioxidants that contribute to overall health. As mentioned above, there are 28 essential vitamins and minerals that play key roles in the body. Phytochemicals are natural bioactive compounds found in plant foods that work with nutrients and dietary fiber to protect against disease. Antioxidants are nutrients that can prevent or slow the oxidative damage to the body, reducing the risk of heart disease, macular degeneration, diabetes, and cancer.

The healthiest carbohydrates to consume are unprocessed whole foods that are high in nutrients, antioxidants, and fiber. These foods raise your blood-sugar levels slowly and minimally. Optimal sources of carbohydrates include *vegetables, fruits, legumes,* and *whole grains.*

Glycemia
Glycemia is a term referring to glucose or sugar in the blood stream. *High-glycemic* foods are those that create a noticeable

rise in blood glucose. These include processed grains (white flour, white rice), sugar (in all of its forms), high-sugar fruits (pineapple, bananas), and starchy vegetables (white potatoes, corn). *Low-glycemic* foods cause a relatively minor elevation of blood sugar. Carbohydrates from this group include low-starch vegetables (broccoli, peppers, leafy greens), low-sugar fruits (berries, apples), and whole grains (steel-cut oats, quinoa).

When you eat high-glycemic food, your blood-sugar levels rise rapidly and then plummet. This means you will be hungry again after a fairly short period of time. You will then find yourself yearning for foods that will raise your blood sugar quickly, which of course means that you'll be craving more high-glycemic carbs. As a result, the more of these foods you eat, the sooner and more often you will feel hungry, and the more intense your cravings will be. It's a vicious cycle.

Moreover, when you eat a lot of high-glycemic foods, your body tends to store more of the food you eat as fat. Your body also becomes more resistant to burning stored fat as fuel. This is due to the workings of the hormone insulin.

Insulin

Insulin is a hormone secreted by the pancreas in response to carbohydrate consumption (and protein, but to a much lesser extent). The job of insulin is to lower blood-sugar levels by guiding your digested food into the cells of the body, where it is either burned as fuel or stored as fat. Some of the carbohydrates you consume will pass into the blood stream as glucose and be transported to the muscles and the brain. Part of the excess sugar will be converted into glycogen and stored in the muscles for later use. The rest will be stored as fat.

When you consume a lot of carbohydrates, especially of the high-glycemic variety, your pancreas has to secrete substantial quantities of insulin to handle the high influx of blood sugar. When there is a large amount of insulin in the bloodstream, your body tends to store food as fat and to hold onto the fat you've already accumulated.

In addition to the health risks involved, a person who is regularly producing large amounts of insulin may eat relatively small amounts of food and still find it very difficult to lose weight. Moreover, this person will be hungrier more often and their cravings will be stronger. As a result, weight loss may feel like an uphill battle.

If you have a history of consuming lots of refined carbohydrates and your body is producing copious amounts of insulin in response, the cells of the body can eventually become insulin-resistant. This means that they lose their ability to respond well to insulin, which can lead to Type 2 diabetes.

Glycemic Index and Glycemic Load

The *glycemic index (GI)* is a numerical system for measuring the rise in blood sugar triggered by a particular food; the higher the number, the greater the blood-sugar response. Therefore, a low GI food will cause a small rise, while a high GI food will trigger a dramatic spike.

The *glycemic load (GL)* is a newer and more precise system. Whereas the GI value tells you only how rapidly a particular carbohydrate turns into sugar, the GL takes serving size into consideration. Carrots, for example, have a high GI. But you'd have to eat about a pound of them before your glucose levels would rise significantly, so a carrot's GL is relatively low.

The GL list can give you a working knowledge of which foods to eat plentifully, moderately, and minimally. Choosing foods that are moderate to low on this list will help you eat more healthfully, feel more satiated, and reduce cravings.

The GL List

Below is an abbreviated list of some typical foods and where they appear on the glycemic load scale.

High-Glycemic Load Foods: Cornflakes, doughnuts, linguini, macaroni, pancakes, rice, russet potatoes

Medium-Glycemic Load Foods: bananas, navy beans, pearl barley, sweet potatoes

Low-Glycemic Load Foods: apples, carrots, chickpeas, grapes, kidney beans, lentils, oranges, pinto beans, pears, red lentils, strawberries, watermelon

For a more complete list, visit *www.mendosa.com/gilists.htm*

Be aware that when you combine a high GL and a low GL food, you change the overall effect of that food on glucose and insulin levels. So, although raisins (or any dried fruit) are a high GL food, mixing them with protein or fat such as nuts will lower the overall effect on glucose and insulin.

Fiber

Low GL foods tend to be higher in fiber than high GL foods. This is good news. Fiber aids in digestion. It can lower cholesterol and slow the absorption of sugar, reducing the risk of Type 2 diabetes. Eating high-fiber foods can also help with weight loss in the following ways:

- They require more chewing time, giving your body time to register the fact that you're no longer hungry and thereby reducing your risk of overeating.
- They help maintain feelings of satiety longer.
- They have more volume for fewer calories.
- They prevent the sharp increases and drops in blood sugar that occur when you consume refined carbohydrates.

Simple Versus Complex Carbohydrates

Carbohydrates are often categorized as simple and complex. Sugars and refined flour products are simple, consisting of only one or two units in each molecule. In contrast, complex carbohydrates are built of chains of simple sugars. They are found in starches such as grains, beans, and vegetables such as squash and potatoes.

Simple carbohydrates are not an optimal choice for weight loss, since they are high-glycemic foods with little nutritional value. However, some complex carbohydrates such as potatoes, (especially baked), are high glycemic,. They will also raise blood sugar and insulin quickly, despite their high fiber and nutrient content.

Consequently, while it's helpful to have a general understanding of simple and complex carbohydrates, the glycemic load index is a better indicator of which food choices are optimal and which should be minimized in your diet.

Protein

Protein is the body's major building material. It is essential to every cell's metabolic activity. The brain, muscles, blood, skin, hair, nails, and the connective tissues that hold the body together are all made mostly of protein. The antibodies of the immune system are constructed of protein, as are all the enzymes and many of the hormones that regulate the body's biochemical activities.

Adequate protein is essential for the development of the fetus, the production of human milk, the height and weight increases of children, the healing of a wound, and the constant growth of hair and nails. It is also needed to replace and maintain body tissues such as muscles, blood, skin, body organs, and connective tissue, all of which are constantly being torn down and rebuilt. In addition, protein is needed in smaller amounts to make enzymes and some of the hormones that regulate the body's processes. It is an important component of the immune system. In addition, it plays an essential role in maintaining the body's water balance. Healthy sources of protein include *meat, poultry, fish, dairy, nuts, beans, legumes, soy products (miso, tamari, tempeh,* and *tofu),* and *whey protein powder.*

Protein and Hormonal Response

Protein has very little effect on glucose or insulin production. In fact, protein consumption initiates the production of another hormone, *glucagon*, the sister hormone of insulin. Whereas insulin is responsible for storing fat, glucagon is in charge of releasing fat from storage and preparing it to burn energy. In other words, insulin is the fat-storing hormone and glucagon is the fat-burning hormone. When these two hormones are in balance, your system will metabolize fat for energy in an efficient manner.

The different roles of insulin and glucagon can be summed up as follows:

Insulin
- Lowers blood-sugar level
- Stores fat
- Is triggered by carbohydrates

Glucagon
- Raises blood-sugar level
- Mobilizes fat from storage
- Is triggered by protein

Including protein in every meal helps to stabilize blood sugar by bringing these two hormones into balance. Moreover, protein takes longer to digest and metabolize than carbohydrates do. Therefore, it makes you feel satisfied for a longer period of time. Because protein (and fat) activate the body's innate satiety mechanisms, including proper amounts of these foods in your eating plan will make you less likely to overeat.

Protein and Muscle Mass

Because protein plays such an important role in building muscle, eating an adequate amount of protein will also help you maintain or even increase muscle mass while losing fat. This is important because muscle is metabolically active. You can raise your metabolism by eating enough protein and engaging in an effective, muscle-building exercise program (explained in Chapter Eight). This will increase the speed and efficiency with which you lose weight, and will help you keep the weight off once you've lost it.

Fat

There is a lot of misunderstanding regarding this macronutrient. It has been demonized and blamed for causing or contributing to a number of health problems, including obesity.

The truth is that we could not live without healthy fat in our diet. Fats are required for hormone production, facilitation of oxygen transport, and the absorption of calcium and the fat-soluble vitamins A, D, E (the premier antioxidant), and K.

Healthy fat is absolutely essential for healthy skin and hair. It slows the aging process. It protects against osteoporosis, arthritis, heart disease, cancer, allergies, and asthma. It lubricates the cell membranes. It also helps cells function optimally so they can fight bacteria and viruses.

Most importantly for weight loss, fat helps to stabilize blood-sugar levels, increase satiety, and decrease cravings.

The Major Sources of Fat

Fats are generally broken up into four categories:

- *Saturated fat* is solid at room temperature. It is found in animal and dairy products. It is also found in vegetable sources such as coconut and palm oil.

- *Monounsaturated fat* is liquid at room temperature. It is found in olives and olive oil, avocados, canola oil, most nuts (including nut oils and nut butters), and seeds (including seed oils and seed butters).
- *Polyunsaturated fat* is also liquid at room temperature. It is found in fish (salmon, tuna, mackerel, etc.), and in vegetable, corn, and soy oils.
- *Trans fats* are solid at room temperature. They are generally artificial fats made by a chemical process called partial hydrogenation. Liquid vegetable oil is packed with hydrogen atoms and converted into a solid fat. Trans fats are found in margarine, vegetable oils, and fried foods. Any processed food with the words "hydrogenated," "partially hydrogenated," or "soy oil" on the ingredient label contains trans fat.

The traditional nutritional advice has been to minimize consumption of saturated fats and ingest primarily poly- and monounsaturated fats. Current scientific studies are reexamining this issue.

Saturated Fat
In February 2010, the very distinguished American Journal of Clinical Nutrition published a landmark study from the Harvard School of Public Health and the Children's Hospital Oakland Research Institute[1] that has turned the current fat recommendation upside down. The conclusion drawn from this study is that "there is no significant evidence for concluding that dietary saturated fat is associated with an increased risk for heart disease."

Coconut oil, in particular, has a number of noted health benefits. It contains lauric acid, an antimicrobial fatty acid that fights bacteria, viruses, and fungi. Some of its surprising benefits include an ability to lower cholesterol, reduce the risk of heart disease, and stimulate weight loss. It has also been found to benefit conditions such as diabetes, chronic fatigue and fibromyalgia, digestive disorders, and thyroid imbalances. As an added plus, it has fewer calories than most other fats—seven calories per gram versus the nine found in most other oils.

Butter, in small amounts, can be beneficial to your health. It contains several important vitamins and minerals, and contains short-chain fatty acids, which don't store easily as body fat. When choosing between butter and margarine (see *trans fats* below), butter wins hands down.

Unsaturated Fat

Monounsaturated Fats are heart-healthy sources. Choose cold-pressed, extra virgin olive oil, cold-pressed or expeller-pressed canola oil, and raw nuts and seeds.

Polyunsaturated Fat is a large class of fatty acids with many members, including both *omega-6s* and *omega-3s*. These fatty acids are the building blocks of hormones and "mini hormones" (called eicosanoids) that control dozens of metabolic processes in the body. If the hormones or mini hormones are not properly regulated, disease results.

Eating balanced amounts of these two fatty acids is extremely important to our health. The ideal fat has somewhere between a 1:1 and a 4:1 ratio of omega-6 to omega-3. The average person eating a Western diet is consuming between 20:1 and 25:1. High rates of omega-6s to omega-3s are associated with increased prostate and breast cancer risk, increased risk of heart disease, and increases in inflammatory and autoimmune diseases.

The problem is made worse by the fact that most of the omega-6s we ingest are unhealthy, coming from highly refined and processed vegetable oils such as safflower, sunflower, soybean, and corn. These oils are very fragile. They break down easily because they are highly processed. To refine them, they are heated to 400 to 500 degrees (trans fats are formed at 320 degrees), bleached, deodorized, and treated with chemical solvents like hexane, a dry-cleaning fluid. All the nutrients are removed in the process. What remains is oil with very little taste, lots of trans fat, and the dangerous potential to create free radicals in the body.

Free radicals occur normally under certain conditions: as part of the metabolic process, when your body creates them to assist the immune system, and also as a result of environmental conditions such as pollution or cigarette smoke. Normally, your body can handle free radicals, but an overabundance can do a lot of damage. They can kill healthy cells, damage your DNA, and accelerate the aging process.

Omega-3 fats protect the heart and the brain, support circulation, boost mood, and lower blood pressure. Most people who eat a Western diet need more omega-3s. *Mackerel, sardines,* and *cold-water fish* such as *wild salmon* are wonderful sources of omega-3s, as are *fish oil supplements. Flaxseeds (and flaxseed oil)* are among the best plant sources.

Trans Fat is made when a manufacturer adds hydrogen to vegetable oil. The purpose of hydrogenation is to increase the flavor, stability, and shelf life of processed foods. Trans fat is found in margarine and shortening, in fried foods like french fries and doughnuts, crackers, and baked items of all kinds. Trans fats are known to increase blood levels of low-density lipoprotein (LDL), or "bad" cholesterol, while lowering levels of high-density lipoprotein (HDL), known as "good" cholesterol. It can also cause major clogging of the arteries and Type 2 diabetes.

To summarize:
- Some saturated fat is good for you.
- Omega-3s are very helpful.
- Monounsaturated fats are beneficial.
- Omega-6s are healthy in limited amounts if they haven't been processed and refined.
- Trans fats are poison to your system.

The Bottom Line

Good fats are naturally occurring, traditional fats that haven't been damaged by high heat, refining, processing, or other industrial tampering, such as partial hydrogenation. The very best of the good fats are found in *fish, nuts, avocados, seeds, coconut,* and surprisingly, *fresh butter. Cold-pressed, extra-virgin olive oil* and *cold-pressed* or *expeller-pressed canola oil* are among your best choices for cooking.

Animal fats should be kept to a minimum because the toxins fed to animals in the form of hormones and antibiotics are stored in their fat. Avoid all fried foods. Avoid refined vegetable oils such as those found in the average supermarket. They oxidize easily and have been processed with high heat and chemicals, which further damage them.

It is important to eat enough fat, since fat is responsible for satiety and stable blood sugar, and "good" fats are an important part of a well-balanced diet. When you don't eat enough fat, you may not feel satisfied with your meal, and are more likely to feel hungry within a short period of time.

Low-fat foods are often higher in sugar than their fattier counterparts. Sugar is the real culprit in such foods. It has no nutritional value and stimulates food cravings. Put away your *PAM* spray and your fat-free salad dressings. Take out the olive oil. Have some almond butter. It will support your weight loss and your health.

Water

The body uses water for virtually all of its functions: digestion, absorption, transporting nutrients, building tissue, and maintaining body temperature. Every cell in the body depends on water to carry out its essential activities. Water in blood plasma, as well as water inside the cells and in the space between the cells, serves as a solvent to transport nutrients to each cell. It also carries waste products from the lungs, kidneys, gastrointestinal tract, and skin for elimination.

Water acts as the climate-control system for the body, maintaining body temperature through perspiration, which then evaporates. It also has wonderful effects on the skin; it plumps it up, fills in lines, balances out oil content, moisturizes dry and dehydrated skin, clears up breakouts, removes toxins, transports essential nutrients to the surface, and increases blood flow, giving your skin color.

In terms of weight loss, water does the following:
- Assists the body in metabolizing stored fat: when your kidneys don't get enough water, the liver has to help them perform. One of the liver's functions is to metabolize fat, and it can't execute this function effectively if it has to do part of the work of the kidneys as well.
- Relieves fluid retention problems: if you don't give your body enough water, it will hold onto what little water it has, thereby causing bloating.
- Reduces fat deposits in the body
- Reduces sodium buildup in the body
- Helps to maintain proper muscle tone
- Contributes to feelings of fullness

It is generally recommended that you drink approximately eight glasses of water per day. Add another eight ounces for every 25 pounds of excess weight you carry.

The Controversy: Low Carb versus Low Fat

For more than three decades, official recommendations have emphasized reduced fat intake along with generous portions of grain consumption as the primary method of achieving and maintaining a healthy body weight. The best estimates regarding nutritional intake in the US indicate that while the percentage of fat in our diets has declined over the past three decades, it has been accompanied by a simultaneous increase in carbohydrate and overall caloric intake. Because of these dietary changes, the number of Americans who are overweight or obese has increased. In addition, diabetes rates have increased and heart disease remains the leading cause of death in most industrialized countries.[2]

The reasons for the expansion of our collective waistlines have been elucidated in previous sections of this chapter. To summarize, an overabundance of easily digested carbohydrates causes blood-sugar spikes, and surges in insulin production. These spikes and surges intensify both hunger and food cravings. They also interfere with your body's ability to use the food you eat as fuel, making the body more inclined to store and retain fat.

The Experts Weigh In

As Dr. Meir Stampfer, a professor of epidemiology and nutrition at the Harvard School of Public Health, states, "It's been the standard advice for decades that Americans should follow lower-fat, high-carb diets. But now it's backfiring. It's clear this doesn't work because it's not as satiating and people just start eating more calories."[3]

In a very provocative article in *Science* (Vol 291, 30 March 2001), entitled "The Soft Science of Dietary Fat," prominent science writer Gary Taubes states: "Mainstream nutritional science has demonized dietary fat, yet 50 years and hundreds of millions of dollars of research have failed to prove that eating a low fat diet will help you to live longer."[4]

Walter Willet, chairman of the department of nutrition at the Harvard School of Public Health, may be the most visible critic of the USDA's low-fat, high-grain recommendations. Willet is the spokesman for the longest running, most comprehensive diet and health studies ever performed, which include data on nearly 300,000 individuals. These data, says Willet, clearly contradict the *low-fat-is-good* health message, and also contradict the idea that all fat is bad for you. He goes on to say that the belief that all fat is harmful may have contributed to the obesity epidemic![5]

The Dietary Intervention Randomized Controlled Trial (DIRECT)[6]

Researchers at Ben-Gurion University of the Negev in Beer Sheva, Israel, and at Brigham and Women's Hospital's (BWH) Channing Laboratory evaluated three different weight-loss diets over two years. They reported the results in the *Journal of Medicine* in July of 2008.

The researchers followed 322 obese patients (mean age 52), who were randomized to either a low-fat, Mediterranean or low-carbohydrate diet for two years.

The low-fat, restricted-calorie diet allowed 1500 calories per day for women and 1800 calories per day for men, with 30% of calories from fat (10% of fat calories from saturated fat), and an intake of 300 mg of cholesterol per day. The participants were asked to consume low-fat grains, vegetables, fruits, and legumes and to limit their consumption of additional fats, sweets, and high-fat snacks.

The Mediterranean diet was a moderate-fat, restricted-calorie diet, rich in vegetables and low in red meat, with poultry and fish replacing beef and lamb. Calories were restricted to 1500 per day for women and 1800 per day for men, with a goal of no more than 35% of calories from fat; primary sources of fat were olive oil and nuts.

The low-carbohydrate, non–restricted-calorie diet aimed to provide 20 grams (approximately 80 calories), of carbohydrates per day for the two-month induction phase, with a gradual increase to a maximum of 120 grams (approximately 360 calories), per day during the maintenance phase. The intake of total calories, protein, and fat was not limited. However, participants were counseled to choose vegetarian sources of fat and protein, and to avoid trans fat.

The results? The average weight loss for the three groups was *6.4 lbs* (2.9 kg) for the *low-fat* group, *9.7 lbs* (4.4 kg) for the *Mediterranean-diet* group, and *10.4 lbs* (4.7 kg) for the *low-carbohydrate* group. (As an interesting aside, women fared better with the Mediterranean diet, while men tended to lose more with the low-carbohydrate diet.)

Another Low-Carbohydrate versus Low-Fat Study

In another recent, albeit much smaller study, leading nutrition researchers, including Dr. Walter Willet and his colleagues, designed an experiment to determine whether low-fat or low-carbohydrate diets were better for losing weight.[7]

For twelve weeks the researchers fed their group of overweight patients three different diets.

1. The first group ate a low-fat diet of 1500 calories for the women and 1800 calories for the men—55% carbohydrates, 30% fat, and 15% protein.

2. The second group ate the same number of calories, but in the form of a low-carbohydrate diet—5% carbohydrates, 65% fat, and 30% protein.

3. The third group also consumed a low-carbohydrate diet, but ate 300 more calories a day than the other two groups.

The results were startling. The low-carbohydrate group eating the same number of calories as the low-fat group actually lost more weight—an average of 23 pounds, compared to 17 pounds for the low-fat group, despite eating the same number of calories. What was even more surprising was that the group eating 300 additional calories a day on the low-carbohydrate diet lost more weight than those eating the low-fat diet—three more pounds per person—than the low-fat group.

What kind of food was consumed? The low-carbohydrate diet was predominantly a diet of whole, unprocessed foods: lean animal protein, vegetables, whole grains, and beans. The low-fat group ate foods that were higher in refined carbohydrates.

Metabolic Syndrome

Emerging research is showing that carbohydrate-restricted diets are an effective strategy not only for weight loss, but for the improvement of Metabolic Syndrome (also known as Insulin Resistance Syndrome, or Syndrome X). This is a cluster of associated health issues that indicate a predisposition to obesity, diabetes, and cardiovascular disease.

Consistent with the idea that intolerance to carbohydrates (insulin resistance) is an underlying feature of Metabolic Syndrome, research has shown that a reduction in dietary carbohydrates results in an overall improvement in the markers associated with this syndrome.

Thus, it appears that carbohydrate-restricted diets are at least as effective as, if not more effective than, low-fat diets for weight loss. They are also associated with improvement in a broad array of cardiovascular risk factors, particularly those related to Metabolic Syndrome.

Dr. Willet and his colleagues have also studied the relationship between glycemic load and carbohydrate intake and the risk of heart disease. They concluded:

"Our findings suggest that a high intake of rapidly digested and absorbed carbohydrate increases the risk of coronary heart disease independent of conventional coronary risk factors. These data add to the concern that the current low-fat, high-carbohydrate diet recommended in the United States may not be optimal for the prevention of coronary heart disease and could actually increase the risk in individuals with high degrees of insulin resistance and glucose tolerance."

Low-Carbohydrate Diets

Low-carbohydrate diets have been vilified by mainstream nutritionists and often misrepresented as "no-carb" diets. This misunderstanding arises from a limited knowledge of how these food plans operate.

Most of these diets are introduced in phases.
1. In the first phase, sometimes referred to as the "induction phase," carbohydrate consumption is very low; all sugar and grains are removed, and sometimes fruit and dairy as well. Protein, fat, and calorie intake are usually not restricted. This phase lasts for two to three weeks.

2. The dieter then moves to a less strict phase, gradually adding carbohydrates back into the diet, choosing the lowest glycemic load foods first. By slowly reintroducing these foods, the dieter can determine the amount of carbohydrates and general food intake he or she can consume while still losing weight.

3. The maintenance phase occurs when the dieter has achieved goal weight. Carbohydrates are slowly increased until the dieter has found the upper limit of carbohydrate consumption that allows for weight maintenance.

The goal of the first phase is to bring the body back into hormonal balance. Blood sugar and insulin levels, food cravings and hunger are reduced, glucagon production increases, and weight loss is usually significant.

The pounds come off more slowly during the second phase—usually one to three pounds per week—as carbohydrates are reintroduced into the diet.

The primary criticism of low-carbohydrate diets arises from ignorance of these various stages. Many critics are only aware of the first and most extreme phase, and base their opinion on this limited knowledge. Obviously a diet of primarily fat and protein will have health repercussions if followed over an extended period of time. However, these food plans are built around progressive stages of increased carbohydrate consumption.

Most low-carbohydrate dieters who adhere to the food plan as intended, and gradually increase their carbohydrate intake while decreasing protein and fat, will eventually find themselves getting about 40% of their calories from (low-glycemic) carbohydrates, 30% from protein, and 30% from fat.

The Food Plan

The percentages mentioned above—40% carbohydrates, 30% protein and 30% fat—are a healthy balance of macronutrients for most people. Some will need more carbohydrates in their diet, and others more fat. We are all different, and as stated earlier in this book, there is no single nutritional plan that will be successful for everyone. Nevertheless, the 40-30-30 approach works for many. Start with those percentages, and adjust as needed. ·

· For an interesting approach to diet that prescribes differing macronutrient percentages based upon your "metabolic type," check out the "Metabolic Typing Diet" proposed by William Wolcott and Dr. Joseph Mercola. It is based on the idea that we all have unique biochemical or metabolic needs and we can tailor our diets in a manner that will effectively support those needs. You can read more about it on Dr Mercola's website at: http://www.mercola.com/2002/dec/18/metabolic_typing.htm

USDA Guidelines

Before 2005, the USDA nutrition guidelines recommended macronutrients in the following proportions:
- Carbohydrates: 55% to 60%
- Protein: 12% to 15%
- Fat: 25% to 30%

The USDA Food Pyramid, and the USDA's new food icon, My Plate, (http://www.choosemyplate.gov/) reflects these recommendations. They emphasize high grain intake and minimal fat consumption.

The updated 2005 Dietary Guidelines for Americans[8] modifies the distribution of nutrients as follows:
- Carbohydrates: 45% to 65%
- Protein: 10% to 35%
- Fats: 20% to 35%

This is a great improvement. It makes room for the *40/30/30* approach endorsed by Dr. Barry Sears, Ann Louise Gittleman Ph.D., and many other earlier proponents of this formula:
- Carbohydrates: 40%
- Protein: 30%
- Fats: 30%

With the 40/30/30 approach, carbohydrate consumption, or more specifically grain and sugar consumption, is reduced, and protein and fat increased. Your main carbohydrate sources are low-glycemic vegetables and a moderate amount of fruit. Some grain is acceptable, but not the six to nine servings previously recommended by the USDA Food Pyramid.· Healthy protein and fat sources are endorsed. The benefits are as follows:

· As an alternative to the USDA's pyramid, faculty members at the Harvard School of Public Health built the Healthy Eating Pyramid. It resembles the USDA's in shape only. The Healthy Eating Pyramid takes into consideration, and puts into perspective,

- You will be less hungry.
- Your cravings will decrease.
- Your body's ability to burn fat will improve.

In addition, insulin resistance will decrease, along with all the other health risks associated with Metabolic Syndrome.

40/30/30 Guidelines
- Choose protein from high-quality sources like eggs, lean meats, poultry, nuts, legumes fish, whey protein powder.
- Eat lots of low-glycemic vegetables and a moderate amount of fruit.
- Don't be afraid of fat. Select from good sources like fish (also high in protein), seeds, nuts, avocados, flaxseed oil, coconut oil, butter, and extra-virgin, cold-pressed olive oil.
- Eat small amounts of "good" starchy carbohydrates like sweet potatoes, oatmeal, lentils, and beans; and whole grains such as whole wheat, brown rice, and bulgur.

How to Eat a 40/30/30 Diet
- Eat three meals a day.
- Include snacks, depending on the amount of time between meals. As a rule, don't go more than four hours without eating. Basically, eat when you are hungry but not starving.
- Eat some protein (two to four ounces), and fat (at least one teaspoon), at each meal.
- Have one to two servings of starchy carbohydrates at each meal. One serving is half a cup or one ounce.
- Allow yourself two to three fruit servings per day.
- Drink one to two glasses of milk a day if you tolerate dairy.
- Eat all the non-starchy vegetables you want.

---

the wealth of research conducted during the last twenty years that has reshaped the definition of healthy eating. Check out this alternative food pyramid at:
http://www.hsph.harvard.edu/nutritionsource/pyramids.html

- Reduce or eliminate sugar and processed carbohydrates.
- Avoid fried foods.
- Drink about eight glasses of water a day.

Meal Ideas

Breakfast
Toasted sprouted wheat bread with peanut butter
Boiled eggs
Filtered water

Vegetable omelet with cheese
Whole-grain bagel
Tea with Stevia

Oatmeal with milk
Raisins
String cheese
Seltzer water

All-Bran cereal
Whey protein and water, mixed
Banana

Fruit Smoothie:
1 c. fresh or frozen fruit (strawberries, raspberries, blueberries, or peaches)
1 scoop of protein powder
8 oz. filtered water
1 tbsp. flaxseed oil
¼ tsp. Stevia Plus to taste

Scrambled eggs with mushrooms and onions
Applesauce, unsweetened

Lunch
Chicken and vegetable soup
Whole-grain crackers
Milk

Vegetable salad with chicken, tuna, or beef
Salad dressing
Seltzer water

Sandwich wrap with chicken or beef, cheese, lettuce, tomato, roasted peppers, and onions
Baby carrots
Vegetable juice

Tuna salad sandwich on sprouted wheat bread
Snow peas and cherry tomatoes

Hamburger
Whole-wheat roll
Tomatoes, lettuce
Sugar snap peas

Beef stew
Roll with butter
Filtered water
Dinner
Chili
Vegetable Salad
Whole-wheat roll
Milk

Roast chicken
Roasted vegetables
Filtered water

Steak kabob with mushrooms, peppers, tomatoes
Corn on the cob
Vegetable salad
Iced tea

Antipasto
Veggie burger on whole wheat bun
Steamed broccoli and cauliflower
Milk

Chicken parmesan—baked, not fried
Roasted peppers and onions
Filtered water

Spaghetti Squash
Tomato sauce
Salmon
Brown rice

Snacks
Apple or banana with almond butter
String cheese and whole wheat crackers
Cottage cheese and fruit
Nuts and dried fruit
Whole wheat bread and cashew butter

The Emotional Aspects of Overeating

Pay Attention to Your Feelings

The 40/30/30 weight-loss plan may be a radically different way for you to eat. You might feel deprived as you eat fewer of your favorite foods. You may also experience emotions such as resentment, sadness, or anxiety. Notice these feelings as they arise. Also, pay attention to any negative beliefs that surface regarding the weight-loss process. You may find yourself thinking that this approach is too difficult, too radical, or too time-consuming. Or you may have doubts that it can actually work for you.

As mentioned in Chapter Two, keeping a journal of thoughts and feelings that arise as you move through this program can be very helpful. Later on, in Chapter Seven, we will explore the use of EFT to work with the negative ideas and emotions that inevitably crop up.

EFT will help you transition successfully from your old eating patterns to this new, healthier way of eating. It will allow you to neutralize any and all uncomfortable emotions or negative beliefs that may come up. With consistent and persistent application of this method, you will be able to make the best food choices, letting go of your weight-loss struggles for good.

CALL TO ACTION

1. Study the "Nutrition Recommendations for Weight Loss" and begin to incorporate these into your diet. You may move toward the 40/30/30 nutritional approach gradually. Or you may wish to try one of the many well-known, low-carb diets, such as Atkins or South Beach.

2. Notice what feelings or negative thoughts come up as you make changes, and jot them down in a journal. In later chapters you will learn to use EFT to neutralize painful feelings and transform unhelpful beliefs.

3. Continue to practice EFT as directed for food cravings, "dangerous times," and general overeating.

4. Continue to listen daily to the hypnosis recording, "Freedom from Excess Weight." or to the recording of your choice (see Appendix).

Chapter Five
FACTORS THAT UNDERMINE
WEIGHT LOSS

In the previous chapter we discussed hormonal responses to food. To recap, an overabundance of processed, easily digested carbohydrates raises insulin levels, causing the body to store food as fat rather than using it for fuel. By decreasing or even eliminating refined carbohydrates in your diet, and by increasing your consumption of vegetables and fruits, whole grains, protein, and healthy fat, you can decrease *insulin*—the *fat storing* hormone—and increase *glucagons*—the *fat burning* hormone. You can bring your body into balance, thus decreasing food cravings, increasing food satiety, and improving your body's ability to burn food for fuel.

There are several other factors that can negatively influence weight loss beside excess consumption of carbohydrates. For example, you may have inherited a body low in certain brain chemicals, predisposing you to sugar addiction. Or you may have an allergic-type reaction to food, causing weight gain due to bloating and uncontrollable food cravings. It is also possible that you are leptin-resistant, making it hard to sense when you've had enough to eat, and increasing your body's propensity to store food as fat instead of using it for fuel. In any of these situations, an over-consumption of refined carbohydrates will cause or exacerbate the problem.

Sugar Sensitivity

Nowhere is the mind/body connection more apparent than in the realm of sugar sensitivity. What you eat strongly impacts blood-sugar levels and certain brain chemicals. These chemicals in turn affect how you feel and act. Consequently, when they consume carbohydrates, people who are sensitive to "the white stuff" experience greater emotional ups and downs than the average person.

Dietician Kathleen DesMaisons, PhD. observes that some people are addicted to sugar in the same way an alcoholic is addicted to alcohol. In fact, strong sugar cravings are common in families of alcoholics. People who are extremely sensitive to sugar may suffer from low blood sugar and low levels of the brain chemicals serotonin and beta-endorphin.

Low Blood Sugar

If you are sugar sensitive, you may have inherited abnormally low blood-sugar levels. If so, your body tends to react to carbohydrate consumption by putting out more insulin than it would if your blood-sugar levels were in a higher, more normal range. The result is a rapid spike and subsequent dip in blood-sugar levels. When this happens, you may find yourself instinctively craving more carbohydrates to raise your blood-sugar levels quickly. Such extreme highs and lows can make you vulnerable to the following:

- Moodiness
- Fatigue/Lack of energy
- Restlessness
- Confusion
- Trouble remembering and concentrating
- Frustration
- Irritability and edginess

In addition, every time your blood sugar spikes, your adrenal glands secrete adrenaline (the hormone that alerts the pancreas to secrete insulin). If the adrenals are repeatedly over-stimulated, they begin to fatigue. Adrenal exhaustion depresses the immune system, making you more vulnerable to illness and disease.

Neurotransmitters: Serotonin and Beta-endorphin

Neurotransmitters are molecules that carry signals between nerve cells (neurons), in the brain. Simply put, they are signaling mechanisms that tell your brain how to respond to certain stimuli, which may include your thought patterns or circumstances in the environment around you. Two neurotransmitters that respond to the consumption of high-glycemic carbohydrates are *serotonin* and *beta-endorphin*.

When *serotonin* levels are ideal, you feel mellow and relaxed, hopeful and optimistic. You have a sense of being at peace with life. You feel creative, thoughtful, and focused. You also have an adequate amount of impulse control, which enables you to "just say no" more easily.

The sugar-sensitive person, however, often suffers from low levels of serotonin, which can cause the following:
- Depression
- Distractibility
- Lethargy
- Inattentiveness
- Low impulse control
- Craving for sweets and other refined carbohydrates

So if your serotonin levels are low or unstable, you may crave refined carbohydrates out of a need to feel better. You may be looking for the mood boost, the sense of optimism and equanimity that serotonin provides. Furthermore, your ability to control the urge to eat is compromised because of the abnormally low levels of the brain chemical that helps resist such urges.

Beta-endorphin acts like a powerful, natural painkiller. It creates a sense of well-being, reduces pain, eases emotional distress, increases confidence, and can even produce a sense of euphoria.

Sugar, like alcohol, causes a release of beta-endorphin. It can make you feel "high" and can reduce both physical and emotional pain. People with normal body chemistry can enjoy a moderate intake of sugar without ill effects. But the brain of the sugar-sensitive person who is low in this neurotransmitter has more beta-endorphin receptors than ordinary people. If you are sugar-sensitive, eating sugar can make you feel and act as if you've been drinking alcohol. Sugar can make you funny, relaxed, silly, talkative, and temporarily self-confident. You feel great and you long to keep feeling that way.

Low levels of beta-endorphin, however, can also make you feel the following:

- Tearful
- Reactive
- Isolated
- Depressed
- Hopeless
- Victimized by others
- More sensitive to pain
- Low in self-esteem
- Hungry for sweets

Therefore, the person who is low in beta-endorphins will naturally crave the foods that will allow him or her to feel relaxed, comfortable, and confident.

If you are sugar sensitive, you need to stabilize your blood-sugar levels and optimize your levels of serotonin and beta-endorphin. The way to accomplish this is by increasing your intake of protein and healthy fats, while decreasing or even eliminating sugar and refined flour products.

For more information, visit Kathleen DeMaison's website, *www.radiantrecovery.com*.

False Fat

"False fat" is a term coined by Dr. Elson Haas. It refers to the bloating, edema, and water retention that is often a result of eating too much of the foods your body is sensitive to. This "false fat" can easily add an extra ten pounds or more of water weight.

Not only that, but eating such foods can contribute to the creation of "real" fat as well, due to resulting food cravings.

Just as hay fever causes swelling in the nasal tissues and eyes, food sensitivities cause "swelling" by sending water to surround food particles that your digestive system is unable to break down properly. This process is just a normal part of the anti-inflammatory response; the body perceives these "undigested" particles as foreign invaders and tries to get rid of them. One resulting symptom is abdominal bloating and water retention.

The body also reacts to food sensitivities by releasing adrenaline and other stress hormones. These stress hormones have important anti-inflammatory properties, and their release makes you feel better at first. But when you "crash" from the adrenaline high, you reach for more of the problematic foods and the cycle begins again. Unfortunately, the very foods that you crave are the ones that spike blood sugar and insulin levels, and thus lead to weight gain.

To make matters worse, you can easily become "addicted" to the foods that are causing the allergic reaction in the first place. This happens because the body releases natural opiates in response to the food causing the reaction. The opiates prevent discomfort, just as the presence of alcohol prevents discomfort in the alcoholic. Remove the food that is stimulating the production of feel-good chemicals, and discomfort begins. Discomfort in this case takes the form of cravings, anxiety, and a kind of "withdrawal."

Serotonin levels also drop when you eat unfavorable foods because serotonin is mostly carried by white blood cells; the same cells used by the immune system to produce a "counter response" to such foods. While those white blood cells are busy responding to food they perceive as a threat, they're less able to deliver serotonin to your brain. As mentioned earlier, low levels of serotonin are linked to cravings, depression, and feelings of general yuckiness. Since sugar and high-carb junk foods raise serotonin levels, those are exactly the ones you crave when you're in low-serotonin mode. It's a vicious cycle, both emotionally and physically.

Furthermore, food sensitivities contribute to other health problems. They interfere with the hormonal balance of the endocrine system, including the thyroid and adrenal glands, making it harder for the body to burn fat. They disturb insulin levels, thus signaling the body to store fat. They decrease energy and contribute to insomnia. They can also cause headaches, joint pain, congestion, heartburn, fatigue, mood swings, and immune dysfunction.

Which foods are we most likely to have allergic-type reactions to? Not surprisingly, the top three are wheat, sugar, and dairy. (The next four on the list are corn, soy, eggs, and peanuts.)

Do you see a pattern here?

Do you have food sensitivities?
If your cravings for certain foods are very intense, you may be sensitive to that food. Take the following quiz to see if your cravings are strong enough to make this possibility likely.

Testing
The simplest way to test for sensitivities is through an elimination diet. Follow these steps:

1. Remove the seven listed foods from your diet for two weeks.

2. At the end of the two weeks, choose one food from the list and consume some of it at each meal for two days. Then remove it from your diet again. Repeat for each listed food.

3. Keep a food diary, recording physical and emotional reactions to each food as you introduce it. Watch for symptoms such as bloating, mood swings, and cravings.

Before you begin the testing process, however, apply EFT for the foods that you crave most and have the hardest time taking out of your diet. It will make the whole process much easier.

If you have been trying to lose weight and nothing you've done so far is working, take the test described above. You may uncover a way to cause a dramatic shift in your body's ability to shed those extra pounds.

For more information regarding false fat, visit Dr.Haas's website: www.elsonhaas.com

Leptin

Leptin is a protein hormone produced by the fat cells. When fat cells are full, they release leptin, which sends a signal to the brain, telling it to stop eating. Leptin also helps the brain determine how much fat to put into storage and how rapidly to metabolize food. Optimal leptin levels reduce hunger, increase fat burning, and reduce fat storage.

Obesity can occur when the brain fails to accurately sense leptin levels, which can cause fat to accumulate and metabolism to slow down. People who are overweight often have too much leptin in their blood, but not enough leptin entering their brain. This is called leptin resistance. It means that fat cells are overproducing leptin, but the brain does not know it.

If you eat a diet high in sugar and grains, the sugar gets metabolized into fat (and is stored as fat in your fat cells), which in turn causes surges in leptin. Over time, if your body is exposed to too much leptin, it will become resistant to it, just as your body can become resistant to insulin.

When you become leptin-resistant, your body can no longer receive the messages telling it to stop eating and burn fat, so you stay hungry. This resistance also causes an increase in visceral fat—the fat that's stored in your belly. The result is a vicious cycle of hunger and fat storage that also increases your risk of heart disease and diabetes.

To treat or avoid leptin insensitivity, eat an adequate amount of protein and healthy fats, while decreasing or eliminating sugar and refined-flour products.

Other Factors

Several other factors can make weight loss especially difficult. These include a low-functioning thyroid, PMS, birth control pills, and certain medications.

Low-Functioning Thyroid

About 25% of women develop or have preexisting thyroid problems by the time they reach menopause. The thyroid, a gland located in your neck, is essential in regulating your metabolism. Low thyroid function is associated with decreased metabolic rate and its corresponding symptoms. Symptoms of hypothyroidism include fatigue, lethargy, weight gain, cold hands and feet, thinning hair, and constipation. Hyperthyroidism, which is the opposite problem, is associated with feeling too warm, trembling hands, heart palpitations/rapid heartbeat, difficulty sleeping, and irritability. Some people lose weight while hyperthyroid; others gain it due to an increased appetite. If you experience any of the aforementioned symptoms, have your thyroid levels checked.

Birth Control Pills

Some birth control pills can cause weight gain by 1.) causing fluid retention and 2.) raising insulin levels. If you find yourself putting on pounds after you start taking the pill, talk to your doctor. A pill with lower estrogen content might be helpful.

PMS

Many women experience weight gain before and during their period. Part of this weight gain is due to fluid retention. In addition, many women experience strong cravings for chocolate and other sweets prior to their periods. Although the reasons for the cravings are unclear, they seem to be related to the drop in serotonin levels that occur at that time.

Eating a diet rich in fruit and vegetables and consuming an adequate amount of protein and fat will help stabilize blood-sugar levels and decrease sugar cravings. Tapping on cravings when they are likely to be most intense can also be immensely helpful.

Medication

Some prescription drugs, especially those taken for depression or anxiety, can contribute to weight gain. Again, the reasons are unclear, but these drugs may increase appetite or cause cravings. Some drugs alter metabolism, causing the body to burn calories more slowly or to store fat. Other medications produce fatigue or shortness of breath, making the person less active. A number of medications can also cause water retention.

If you suspect that a medication is causing you to gain weight, talk to your doctor. You may be advised to stop taking the medication, switch to one not associated with weight gain, or take a lower dose. But don't discontinue a medication without first talking to your doctor. Keeping your blood pressure, diabetes, or depression under control is more important than the few excess pounds that may be associated with a particular drug.

CALL TO ACTION

1. Absorb the information contained in this chapter. Research these subjects further if any of the issues described apply to you. Talk to your doctor if appropriate.

2. Continue paying attention to feelings or negative thoughts that come up as you make changes. Write about them in your journal.

3. Continue to practice EFT as directed for food cravings and for times when you are most likely to be tempted to overeat or to make poor food choices.

4. Continue to listen daily to the hypnosis recording, "Freedom from Excess Weight," or to the recording of your choice. (See appendix. You may find the hypnosis recording of "Eat, Drink, and Be Healthy" especially helpful.)

Chapter Six
THE EXCHANGE SYSTEM FOOD PLAN

Often weight loss occurs simply by minimizing the consumption of junk food and making healthier food choices. Cravings decrease and the body becomes more efficient at burning calories. However, calories do count, and if you are still eating too much food, you will not lose weight, no matter how healthy the food you are eating. When general guidelines regarding food choices don't cause weight loss, it becomes necessary to look at how much you are eating, and to learn how to consume less while still eating in a balanced and healthy way.

This chapter will introduce the Exchange System, a system of nutritional units that allows a person to make substitutions within a group of foods without altering the total number of calories and nutritional composition of a diet.

The Exchange System allows you to substitute one food for another without having to do any calculations. For example, you can easily replace one exchange unit of beef for one of chicken or fish. The units have the same caloric content and nutritional composition (more or less), so substituting won't affect the diet's expected benefits.

The Exchange System classifies food into six categories: fruit, vegetables, starchy carbohydrates, protein, fat, and milk. Within each category, there are "exchange equivalents."

How Much Can I Eat?

There are many formulas available to predict exactly how much food you need to eat in order to lose weight. However, losing weight is unpredictable because too many variables can affect the rate at which you will lose weight—factors such as metabolism, muscle mass, age, genetics, amount of exercise, etc.

Nevertheless, here is a formula that will give you a ballpark figure for the number of calories you can ingest and still lose weight:

*For fat loss, consume 12 to 13 calories
per pound of body weight*

*(Maintenance = 15 to 16 calories per pound
of body weight)*

Use this calculation as a guideline only. In the next chapter you will learn how to estimate the amount of food you need by paying attention to hunger and satiety signals, eating only when you are hungry and stopping when you are satisfied. Once you become competent in this skill, you can accurately and intuitively assess how much food you need to consume in order to lose weight while meeting your energy requirements.

Type of Exchange	1400 kcal	1600 kcal	1800 kcal	2000 kcal
Vegetable	3 to 5	3 to 5	3 to 5	3 to 5
Fruit	3	3	3	3
Starchy Carbs	3	4	5	6
Protein	11	12	13	14
Fat	3	4	5	6

Food Exchanges

The chart above indicates approximately how many exchange units you can eat from each food group in order to lose weight in a healthy and balanced manner.

Serving sizes:

Starchy carbohydrates: One exchange is one slice of bread, ½ cup of rice, pasta, corn or beans, one small potato, and one ounce of cereal or crackers.

One starch exchange contains about 15 grams of carbohydrates, 3 grams of protein, a trace of fat, and 80 calories.

Fruit: One exchange is usually one piece of fruit or ½ cup of chopped fresh fruit.

One fruit exchange contains about 15 grams of carbohydrates and 60 calories.

Vegetables: One exchange is one cup of raw vegetables or ½ cup cooked vegetables.

One vegetable exchange contains about 4 grams of carbohydrates, 2 grams of protein, and 25 calories.

Protein: One exchange is equivalent to one ounce of meat, poultry, or fish. It is also equivalent to one egg, ½ cup of beans, one ounce of cheese, or ¼ cup of cottage or ricotta cheese.

One protein exchange contains 7 grams of protein, averages 4 grams of fat, and has an average total of 65 calories.

The calories in protein servings vary widely because of the range in fat content. Lean sources of protein have almost no fat and about 30 calories per exchange. High-fat protein sources contain up to eight grams of fat and over 100 calories per exchange. For the sake of simplicity, the system presented here presumes an average of 65 calories and four grams of fat per exchange.

Fat: One serving is equivalent to one teaspoon of butter or oil, one tablespoon of salad dressing, ½ tablespoon of peanut butter, or 10 peanuts.

One serving contains about 5 grams of fat and 45 calories.

What About Milk?

The original Food Exchange List put forth by the American Dietetic Association listed milk as its own exchange group. However, I don't see this as a necessary choice. As I stated in Chapter Three, an estimated 70% of the world's population is lactose-intolerant. Since you can easily get calcium from other food sources and supplements, I recommend that you drink milk if you like it and tolerate it well, but omit if you don't.

If you do drink milk, here is where it fits into the Food Exchange system:

One 8-ounce glass of 1% milk contains about 2 grams of fat, 12 grams of carbohydrate, 8 grams of protein, and 100 calories. Count this as one protein exchange and half a starchy carbohydrate exchange. 2/3 cup whole milk also has about 100 calories. Count it the same way.

Yogurt

Yogurt is a different story. Many people who have trouble digesting milk have no problem with yogurt. The live cultures promote digestive health, and it is a great source of calcium.

One ¾ cup of plain yogurt made with 1% skim milk or 2/3 cup made with whole milk has about 100 calories, and can be counted as one protein exchange and half a starchy carbohydrate exchange.

A list of food exchanges can be found in the Appendix.

Keep it Simple

Before you start making yourself crazy trying to figure out what and how much you can eat each day, review the guidelines for creating a healthy 40/30/30 meal plan.
- Eat three meals a day.
- Eat some protein (two to four ounces or protein ex-

changes) and fat (at least one teaspoon) at each meal.

- Have one to two servings of starchy carbohydrates at each meal. One serving is a half-cup or one ounce.
- Allow yourself three fruit exchanges per day.
- Eat lots of non-starchy vegetables.
- Reduce or eliminate sugar and processed carbohydrates.
- Avoid fried foods.
- Drink about eight glasses of water a day.

Basically you just need to figure out how much protein and how many starchy carbohydrates you can eat at each meal and snack. Avoid fried foods, cook with a reasonable amount of oil (usually about two tablespoons), and use a sensible amount of butter on cooked veggies (approximately one teaspoon over a cup of cooked veggies), and salad dressing (two tablespoons over two cups of mixed raw veggies). The food plan hasn't changed—only the quantities of some foods have.

To get an idea what this might look like, examine the two food plans that follow.

1400 calories	1800 calories
Breakfast	**Breakfast**
2 scrambled eggs	2 scrambled eggs
1 tsp. Butter	1 tsp. butter
½ banana	½ banana
1 slice whole wheat toast	1 slice whole wheat toast
8 oz. Milk	8 oz. milk
Lunch	**Lunch**
3 oz. Chicken	4 oz. chicken
2 c. vegetable salad	3 c. vegetable salad
1 tbsp. salad dressing	2 tbsp. salad dressing
	1 oz. roll

Snack	Snack
1 apple	1 apple
Dinner	**Dinner**
4 oz. tuna steak	5 oz. tuna steak
½ c. sweet potato	1 c. sweet potato
½ c. broccoli	1 c. broccoli
½ c. carrots	1 c. carrots
1 tsp. butter	2 tsp. butter
½ c. blueberries	½ c. blueberries
2/3 c. yogurt	2/3 c. yogurt

Breakfast is the same for both lists. The 1400-calorie lunch consists of three ounces of chicken, two cups of salad, and one tablespoon of salad dressing. The 1800–calorie lunch has four ounces of chicken, three cups of salad, two tablespoons of salad dressing and one 1-ounce roll. The 1400-calorie snack and the 1800 are the same. For dinner, the 1400-calorie plan includes four ounces of tuna steak, a half-cup of sweet potato, one cup of cooked vegetables, one teaspoon of butter, and yogurt with blueberries. The 1800-calorie meal includes five ounces of tuna steak, one cup of sweet potato, one and a half cups of cooked veggies, and yogurt with blueberries.

Remember that these are guidelines; you don't need to follow them to the letter. Be flexible. Your sense of satiety and your energy levels also need to inform the process.

The 90/10 Rule

Aim to eat well approximately 90% of the time. Occasionally you might choose to treat yourself to something that is not on your food plan. This will not be a problem if it is fueled by *conscious choice* and not *mindless compulsion*.

With a regular EFT practice you will be able to neutralize your food cravings and the anxiety that fuels them. This will create the space for choice.

Food Log

It is a very good idea, at least in the beginning, to have a daily food plan. It can be helpful to know what you intend to eat for each meal and snack. If you don't have a plan, you may spend much of your day thinking about when and what your next meal or snack will be, which will only fuel your compulsion to eat when you are not really hungry.

Look at your plan as a guide to healthy, appropriate eating, but be flexible and open to change when needed. Get familiar with the foods on the exchange list so that you can make substitutions when necessary. You will find a food log you can download on the "**Resources**" page of my website:
www.tlcweightloss.net/resources.php

As You Proceed...

Many people feel relieved when they are finally given "diet" guidelines. They feel that at last they know how much they can eat. While these guidelines can be very helpful, it is important to remember that ultimately this process is about eating intuitively. It is about checking within to see if you are really physically hungry, or are just looking for comfort, distraction, or a way to stuff down your feelings.

We will discuss the practice of paying attention to hunger and fullness at length in Chapter Seven. Meanwhile, remember that while the exchange system provides guiding principles for what and how much to eat, these are not hard and fast rules. You are still responsible for investigating, honoring, and working with the thoughts and feelings that have been driving you to overeat.

CALL TO ACTION:

1. Begin to incorporate the exchange system into your eating plan if it seems appropriate for you.

2. Continue to notice what feelings come up as you make changes in your diet.

3. Continue to practice EFT for food cravings, "dangerous" times, and general overeating.

4. Continue to listen daily to the hypnosis recording, "Freedom from Excess Weight," or to the recording of your choice. (See Appendix.)

Chapter Seven
MINDFUL EATING

To lose weight and keep it off, you need to eat only when you are physically hungry and stop when you have had enough. This requires the successful recognition of hunger and fullness signals and the ability to discern physical versus emotional hunger. You can develop this awareness by *slowing down, turning inward,* and *paying attention.*

Developing the skill of mindfulness will help you:
* Develop awareness of hunger and satiety signals.
* Differentiate between physical and emotional hunger.
* Identify the feelings behind emotion-driven overeating.
* Reduce the stress that prompts overeating.

Developing this type of awareness takes practice, perseverance, and patience. Years of operating on automatic will not abate quickly or effortlessly. But the rewards go far beyond the ability to reign in overeating. It spills over into the rest of your life so that you can be more present, alive, appreciative, and at ease.

You will also learn how to use EFT to neutralize the feelings that prompt you to eat when you are not physically hungry. This is an extremely helpful tool to have. Tapping can create a sense of ease that removes the compulsion to overeat and replaces it with the ability to choose whether you will eat or abstain.

Mindful Consumption

Shedding excess pounds requires eating enough food to maintain your daily energy levels, no more and no less. This means you don't eat to excess, but you don't let yourself starve, either. Although in Chapter Four you were directed to calculate how many calories would probably sustain you and still allow you to lose weight, the number you came up with was only a rough estimate.

How much do you need to eat in order to maintain your energy level and still lose weight? The best way to figure that out is to follow two rules:

Eat when you're hungry;
Stop when you're full.

Simple? Yes. Easy? No.

Physical vs. Emotional Hunger

Develop the habit of questioning your urge to eat. Are you truly hungry, or are you turning to food for other reasons, such as comfort, reward, or distraction?

To clarify what you are feeling, try creating some space between your desire to eat and the eating process itself. When you find yourself thinking about food, pause for a moment. Take a deep breath. Tune into your physical and emotional state.

If you are not physically hungry, what are you feeling? The following is a partial list of uncomfortable feelings you may be trying to anesthetize with food:

anger, anxiety, boredom, emptiness, fear, frustration, guilt, loneliness, loss, resentment, sadness, shame

Watch for patterns. With practice, you will learn to make the connection between a strong urge to eat when you are not hungry and the emotional uneasiness that prompts that urge.

Using EFT to Make Choices

Once you have named your feelings, you can use EFT to defuse them. EFT is a very effective technique for neutralizing emotional distress. If you are in the troughs of a strong, emotionally driven food craving, follow these simple steps.

1. Tune into your emotional state. Identify the feeling and measure the level of its intensity using the SUD scale.

2. Tap on the Karate Chop Point using a Set-Up phrase such as:

    "Even though I feel _____, I deeply and completely accept myself."

3. Move through the sequence of points, using a reminder phrase such as

    "This _____ feeling."

4. Reassess. Check the intensity of your feelings after each round of tapping and continue until the intensity is a two or lower.

Now tune into your desire to eat. Is it still present? Has it decreased? Has it changed in any way? Have other feelings come up? Stay present and observe.

Aspects

Sometimes several feelings may be clustered together. These different feelings are just different *aspects* of the same issue. If, as you tap, you notice another feeling come up that is different from the original, it means that the intensity of the original feeling has subsided enough for a related feeling to arise. You are dealing with another facet of the problem. Simply tap on that feeling until it too subsides.

For example, you might find yourself angry with someone. As you tap, your anger might give way to fear. Tune into the fear, note the intensity, and tap. As you continue to tap, your fear might recede, and feelings of sadness might wash over you. This shifting is quite common. Just keep tapping on each emotion until it has abated, and you feel calm and stable.

Tapping on Physical Discomfort
You can also tune into physical sensations. Is there bodily discomfort that corresponds to the emotions? Where do you feel it? How would you describe it? Is there a heaviness in your chest? A tightness in your throat? Butterflies in your stomach? You can tap on those physical sensations as well.

"Even though I feel this heaviness in my chest…"

"Even though I'm having trouble taking a deep breath…"

"Even though my throat feels tight…"

"Even though I have butterflies in my stomach…"

Be aware that physical sensations, just like emotions, can change. The quality and intensity may shift. They can also move to a different part of the body. A headache at the temple can move toward the back of the head. A stomach pain can move up toward the chest. If this happens, you "chase the pain." Note where the pain has moved to, watch for any changes in the quality or intensity of the sensation, and tap again.

To Eat or Not to Eat
When you have tapped your emotional and/or physical distress down to a two or lower, and have returned to a state of equilibrium, reassess your desire to eat. The strong pull to eat has probably been reduced or erased.

If it hasn't, check within and reassess your physical and emotional state. Repeat the tapping sequence for any discomfort that may still be present.

When your strong impulse to eat has subsided, take another deep breath. From this place of calmness and ease you can decide whether you wish to eat or not. You have moved from compulsion to choice.

Replacing Compulsion with Choice

The purpose of this tapping procedure is to bring you back to a state of equilibrium. You are not tapping to avoid eating. You are tapping to feel better, calmer, and less stressed. Then the eating compulsion can pass. From this place of calm, you can choose whether or not to eat.

This is an important distinction. If you think you have to force yourself to tap to keep from eating something you really want, you may refuse or "forget" to tap.

The purpose, then, is to bring a sense of control to an impulse that once felt uncontrollable. When you have decreased or eliminated your emotional distress, you will recover the ability to make choices.

Occasionally, you may elect to eat the food that prompted you to tap. Remember the *90/10 rule* and aspire to eat well about 90% of the time.

With that said, know that you may pay a price later for a sugar/flour indulgence. If you are sugar sensitive, or have an addictive response to high-glycemic foods, cravings may intensify in the hours and/or days following consumption of such foods. You need to be aware of this possibility. Learn to connect cravings for refined carbohydrates and recent food choices. Then let that knowledge inform your choices in the future. Some people can have a little bit of chocolate or the occasional plate of pasta without after-effects, and some cannot. The only way you will know is by paying attention to what happens in your body.

To Summarize

When you feel the urge to eat, follow these five steps:

1. Pause and take a deep breath.

2. Tune into your emotional state. What do you feel? How strong is the feeling?

3. Tap on the feeling until it has been neutralized.

4. Tune into your body and see if there is a corresponding physical discomfort. If there is, tap until that too has been negated.

5. When you arrive at a state of calmness and ease, you may choose to eat or not.

But I Don't Know How I Feel!

Sometimes you may find it difficult to tell what you feel. In that case, you can use a Set-Up phrase like this:

"Even though I don't know how I feel..."

One of the gifts of EFT is an increase in your intuitive abilities. The wall between the conscious and unconscious becomes more permeable. Tapping on "I don't know how I feel" can create clarity that allows you to more easily identify your emotions.

But even if you can't figure out what the feeling is, the tapping can still produce a sense of ease and relief.

Another option when you cannot name a feeling is to tune into bodily sensations. Physical discomfort is often much easier to identify than buried emotions. If you notice any physical unease, tap until it dissolves. You will notice that your corresponding emotional distress also dissipates.

Developing Awareness

You may find the practice of making connections between feelings and cravings difficult in the beginning. It may not even occur to you to tap until you've already overeaten. Be gentle with yourself. Respect the strength of your compulsion. You may need to work backwards. If you realize you've overeaten without awareness, look back and try to figure out what prompted you to eat; what emotions were driving you. Be curious. As you engage in this inquiry, your ability to recognize the feelings that precede a binge will increase. Think of it as building an awareness muscle.

You may resist identifying your eating triggers because doing so makes you more alert to feelings of shame and remorse—of thinking that you have been "bad." Take this opportunity to neutralize guilt and increase self-acceptance. You can do this by tapping on one or more of the following phrases.

> *"Even though I feel so guilty about eating _____,*
> *I deeply and completely love, accept, and forgive myself."*
>
> *"Even though I feel awful…"*
>
> *"Even though I was bad and I don't know what's wrong with me…"*
>
> *"Even though I know better, I'm so stupid…"*

If you are finding it difficult to pause before the binge begins, you might want to ease into this practice by tapping regularly throughout the day as a preventive measure. You could use one or more of these statements:

"Even though I always want to eat and I can't stop myself; I feel so hopeless..."

"Even though my eating is out of control and I feel (awful, guilty, bad, stupid)..."

"Even though I want to eat_____ whenever I feel_____..."

Getting Help
If you are not getting the results you need, or if the compulsion is greater than your ability to change on your own, get help. Although you can do lots of effective work by yourself, sometimes the aid of an experienced EFT practitioner can be extremely beneficial.

You can contact me at my email address, *terry@tlcweightloss.net*, for a free, 30-minute consultation. During that time I can answer any questions that have come up as you worked through this program and we can decide if more sessions would be helpful.

You can also peruse the list of qualified practitioners at EFT Universe: *www.practitioners.eftuniverse.com/referralMain.aspx*

Moving Through the Process
Using EFT to work through the emotional aspects of overeating is a skill that takes time to master. Much of your eating has probably been unconscious up until now, and old habits die hard.

We all have very good reasons for doing what we do, but unless you are inquisitive, you will never discover what those reasons are. And if you don't know what they are, it will be difficult to make long-lasting changes in your behavior.

Let your food cravings be a guide pointing toward your own healing. When you experience strong food cravings, make a commitment to turn within and examine your feelings. Tap to neutralize those feelings and to bring yourself back to the state of balance and peace that makes conscious choice possible.

Be gentle and kind toward yourself during this process of self-discovery. And remember, if beating yourself up were at all helpful in moving you toward your weight-loss goals, you'd be thin as a rail by now!

Mindful Awareness of Hunger and Satiety

If, upon questioning the nature of your appetite, you discover that you are physically hungry, your next step is to determine just how hungry you are.

On the following page is a hunger/satiety scale that describes the various stages of hunger and fullness and what they feel like. Your goal is to eat when you are fairly hungry, but not starving—about a three on this scale—and to stop when you are comfortably full—about a six.

Do your best to avoid getting really hungry (a one or two). If you eat when your hunger feels out of control, you will be inclined to grab the foods that take the least amount of time to prepare and that raise your blood-sugar levels the quickest. At best you'll grab a bagel, and at worst you'll gravitate toward the cookie jar. Furthermore, you will eat quickly, gobbling down those goodies and stuffing yourself before you've had a chance to really know when you've had enough.

THE HUNGER AND SATIETY SCALE

1 Weak with hunger
You are so hungry that you may not even be aware of it, but you feel headachey and faint.

2 Famished
Too hungry. This is the fist-banging stage when you'll eat anything.

3 Hungry
The perfect time to eat, when the food tastes delicious, but you're not so hungry that you're indiscriminate.

4 Mildly hungry
Something light would suffice, or you could stand to wait another hour for the desire to develop more fully.

5 On the way to being satisfied
During a meal, you are in the pleasant stage of enjoying the food but you are not yet satisfied.

6 Satisfied.
The perfect time (according to your stomach) to stop eating. You are sated.

7 A little fuller than "satisfied."
A few bites past *"6,"* due to the momentum of eating. The food seems less delicious, more tasteless.

8 *Very full*
Beginning to be uncomfortable.

9 Painfully full.

10 And so on.

Trust Your Hunger

If you have been on the dieting roller coaster of starve and binge, you may mistrust your body's hunger signals, afraid that if you give into them you will overeat. And it may be very challenging to discern the difference between real physical hunger and the irresistible pull of food cravings.

You may also be used to eating because food is in front of you, because it is mealtime, or because everyone else is eating. If you have been dieting, you may also be in the habit of starving yourself in an effort to be "good."

Eat when you are hungry, and honor your body's hunger signals. Eating when you are hungry is not what causes you to gain weight. Starving yourself will never lead to permanent weight loss.

Hunger is natural, instinctive, and ultimately trustworthy. Infants and young children innately respond to hunger signals. People who can no longer recognize true hunger need to relearn what they knew as babies. Befriend your appetite. Your body will tell you when you need to eat and when you've had enough. When you eat from body hunger, you develop trust and confidence in your ability to care for yourself.

Overeating

You may struggle with eating too much, despite feelings of fullness. Perhaps you do not want to stop eating because the food "tastes so good." Needing to eat past a point of "enoughness" is probably more about how food makes you feel. Eating can have a soothing and calming effect.

Pay attention to resistance to ending your meal. And then tap.

"Even though I don't want to stop eating…"

"Even though I need to keep eating because I'll feel awful if I stop…"

"Even though I can't get enough..."

Physical Causes of Overeating
Remember that overeating is not always emotion-driven. As mentioned in Chapter Five, the inability to discern feelings of hunger and fullness can be caused or exasperated by leptin resistance. Diet can and usually does influence eating behavior and it is important to pay attention to both.

Think Ahead
Eating well takes planning. Know when and what you will eat each day. Keeping a food journal, as suggested in Chapter Six, can be very helpful. Write your food plan for the day *in pencil,* and re-write it if you choose to replace one food exchange for another. You can use the Food Log found on the Resources page of my website: *www.tlcweightloss.net/resources.php*

As previously stated, extreme hunger can sabotage your best intentions. Arm yourself with portable foods that you can eat when you are hungry, such as fruit, nuts, and cheese.

<u>Mindful Eating</u>

The practice of mindful eating allows you to enjoy your meal with total satisfaction. The more you pay attention to and savor your food, the less likely you are to overeat.

This is often a welcome change for veteran dieters who have been following stringent food plans without regard to hunger, satiety, or personal satisfaction. It may feel like a paradox, but tuning into the pleasure of eating is one of the most helpful practices you can develop for managing your weight.

MINDFUL EATING

1. Sit down in a designated eating place, with as few distractions as possible.

2. Before you eat, observe how your food looks and smells. Acknowledge how fortunate you are for the abundance of food before you. The practice of saying grace before meals, if you are so inclined, can enhance this sense of appreciation and gratitude.

3. Eat slowly and mindfully, noticing the taste and textures of the food you are eating, and savor each mouthful.

4. Put your utensil down between bites.

5. Taking about 20 minutes to eat a meal is optimal, since it takes about that long for the brain to register that the stomach is full. Extend mealtime by pausing momentarily every few minutes. If you can't allow that much time for your meal, be sure that 20 minutes have passed from the time you began eating and the time you reach for seconds. At that point you will know if you really need more food.

6. Become aware of when you have had enough. Observe the sense of fullness in your stomach, and notice that the food you are eating does not taste quite as good as it did when you were hungry.

Mindfulness Practices

The ability to recognize hunger and fullness signals, to discern the difference between physical and emotional hunger, to name and stay present to your thoughts and feelings, and to remain attentive throughout the eating process, can be greatly aided by practices such as meditation and yoga. Regular participation in these methods will assist you in acquiring the skills of mindfulness that are so beneficial to losing weight. They can also help you replace self-criticism with kindness and non-judgment.

In addition, these practices can increase your sense of equanimity. As feelings of calmness increase, you will feel less stressed, and less easily rocked by everyday pressures. Consequently, you will be less likely to respond to the challenges of the day by overeating. Coming into a place of deep stillness on a regular basis will reduce your need to soothe or calm yourself with food.

Over time, these practices can provide a direct connection to your personal sense of spirituality. They can cultivate the understanding that you are not your thoughts, your ideas, or your desires. You learn at a deep level that who you are is unchanging, unique, dear, and precious; not a transitory state.

Below is a brief description of meditation and yoga practices. Meditation techniques and yoga styles are rich and varied. See the Appendix for websites and books that can help you explore this topic further.

Meditation

Meditation is a technique that encourages single-pointed attention. It does this by narrowing your focus to your breath, a sound, an object, or a mantra. It requires a willingness to come back to the object of meditation over and over. No matter how often and how far your mind wanders—and it will wander—you return to your breath, your bell, your candle flame, your prayer.

Counting Breath Meditation

The following is a very simple meditation technique. It involves paying attention to your breath, counting each exhalation.

Start by getting into a sitting position that allows you to be comfortable while maintaining a straight spine.

Next, bring focus to your breath. Begin counting your exhalations. Inhale. Then when you exhale, think "one." Inhale again, and when you exhale this time, count "two." Keep counting silently to yourself until you get to ten. After you reach ten, start over again with "one."

Try to keep the count, but if you lose track, start over at "one." Give your full attention to the count. If you have stray thoughts, notice them and then let them go. Return to counting. Don't intentionally alter your breathing pattern, but let your breath find its own pace and depth, the way a stream finds its course.

Mantra

A mantra is a word or phrase repeated continuously. It may be completely meaningless, or hold some special significance for you. It can be in your native language or in a foreign language. Some words that are often used as mantras are:

- Peace
- Shalom
- Amen
- Ham Sah (Sanskrit for *I Am That*)
- Om

To begin, sit comfortably with your eyes closed and your spine reasonably straight. Repeat the mantra gently in your mind, at whatever tempo feels natural. There is no need to synchronize the mantra with your breathing, but if this occurs naturally, that's fine. Just allow the mantra to arise in your mind, effortlessly.

If and when you notice that your attention has drifted, simply note it and gently begin repeating your mantra again.

Yoga

Yoga is a system of physical postures, breathing techniques, and meditation. In the United States we are most familiar with the postures, or *asanas*. When you work with yoga poses, you combine breath with movement, planting yourself solidly in the body and using gentle physical motion to move into stillness. It is a marvelous practice that can complement your weight-loss efforts in a number of ways.

Moving through the *asanas* grounds you physically, helping you to develop awareness of and trust in your body's needs.

As you practice, you constantly tune into your level of comfort so that you know when to move deeper into a pose and when to back off. It is therefore a method of self-care, giving you permission to nurture yourself. Since self-care is a cornerstone of any long-lasting weight-loss program, yoga can be an invaluable addition to your weight-loss efforts.

Yoga is also a great practice for developing an awareness of your harsh inner critic. Once you are aware of this judgmental voice, you can practice letting it go. Over time, compassion and forgiveness will replace self-criticism.

There are many styles of yoga, and many approaches to teaching it. If you feel drawn to yoga, try a few different classes so that you can find the style that feels right to you.

CALL TO ACTION:

1. Practice developing awareness of a) the feelings that drive overeating and b) the physical sensations that accompany these feelings. Tap on these feelings till they dissolve, using the EFT instructions provided. Then choose whether you really want to eat if you are not physically hungry.

2. Practice using the Hunger/Satiety Scale. Eat when you are at a 3—moderately hungry. And stop when you are comfortably full—around a 6.

3. Practice mindful eating. Eat slowly, with awareness, eliminating as many distractions as possible. Bring full attention to your eating. Do this at least once a day.

4. If inclined, explore and develop a regular mindfulness practice such as meditation or yoga.

5. Continue to listen daily to the hypnosis recording, "Freedom from Excess Weight." or to the recording of your choice. (See Appendix. You may find the "Mindful Eating" recording especially helpful.)

106 *Waist Management*

Chapter Eight
BLOCKS TO SUCCESS

In the previous chapter you learned to use EFT for emotions that prompt overeating. By working with the feelings that arise with your desire to overeat, you can diffuse those feelings. This will allow you to replace compulsion with choice. And as long as you can *choose* to eat well most of the time, you will inevitably reach your goal weight.

The emotions that fuel the desire to overeat are one of the roadblocks that may have sabotaged your weight-loss efforts in the past. Learning to recognize and diffuse these feelings takes practice. Be patient with yourself.

In this chapter you will explore other obstacles that can appear as you move through the weight-loss process. Do your best to meet these hindrances with curiosity and compassion. They are an inevitable part of your weight-loss journey. If this were not so, you would have lost weight with the first diet you tried, and would have kept the weight off effortlessly.

Resisting the Process

The only predictable thing about resistance is that it will emerge, sooner or later. It has appeared when you've tried other weight-loss programs, and it probably will with this one. But instead of doing battle with food and with yourself, you now have an incredibly powerful tool to neutralize the feelings that fuel your struggle—EFT.

Just as you used EFT to neutralize feelings that drove you to overeat, so will you use this technique to diffuse the feelings that fuel your resistance to the weight-loss process.

Feelings That Fuel Resistance

You may be aware of inner conflict about the eating guidelines presented thus far. Here are some feelings that may have arisen, along with EFT statements that might express how you feel. If you identify with any of these feelings, check within to see how strong the feeling is, and give it a number on the SUD scale. Use one of the Set-Up statements provided, or create one that better reflects your emotions.

Deprivation

"*Even though I feel deprived without my favorite foods…*"

"*Even though I feel deprived because I can't eat _____…*"

Sadness

"*Even though I feel so sad when I think that I have to give up_____…*"

Resentment

"*Even though I resent having to be so disciplined when everyone around me is eating whatever they want…*"

Anger

"*Even though it ticks me off that I have to work so hard at this…*"

"*Even though I get so mad that I can't eat what I want…*"

Rebelliousness

"*Even though I don't want anyone telling me how to eat…*"

"Even though I don't want to tap every day, and no one can make me..."

Impatience

"Even though I don't have the patience to eat slowly..."

"Even though I don't have time to create a food plan..."

Fear of Changing Eating Habits

Maybe you are afraid that when you stop overeating, the emotional pain you have been avoiding will emerge. You may feel that you will no longer be able to soothe, comfort, or distract yourself with your favorite foods. You may be afraid that you will not be able to cope with the emotional discomfort—the anxiety, stress, loneliness—and life will be too difficult. What will you think about if you are not constantly focused on food?

"Even though my life will be too difficult or too painful without my favorite foods..."

"Even though I can't possibly cope with the stress in my life if I can't eat what I want..."

"Even though I don't want the pressure of maintaining my weight loss..."

Think about your favorite comfort food, and imagine how you would feel if you could never have it again.

"Even though I feel so anxious when I think about never having _____ again..." (insert a favorite comfort food)

What trauma/feeling/problem are you ignoring by constantly thinking about food?

"Even though I'd have to look closer at my relationship with _____ if I stopped stuffing myself with food..."

"Even though I would have to feel the pain (anger, sadness, shame, loss, guilt) that I've been stuffing down with food..."

"Even though I'm afraid to look at my past..."

If you are dealing with the effects of a painful past and have been using food to cope with the resulting sorrow or anguish, your apprehension is understandable and legitimate. Healing is possible, however. Exploring and healing the past will be covered extensively in the next chapter. For now, be aware of your fear and tap to relieve any sense of dread or anxiety that may crop up.

Fear of Being Thinner

You may be afraid of being thinner for any or all of the following reasons:

1. You fear that if you lose weight you will become more physically and/or sexually attractive and that might be dangerous.

2. Other people in your life may feel threatened or jealous if you lose weight. This could be a spouse, friend, significant other, or family member.

3. Being thinner will feel unfamiliar and uncomfortable.

4. You won't be able to blame all your problems on your weight.

Here are some phrases that might resonate with your fear of being thinner.

"Even though I don't want to be noticed by men/women..."

"Even though it's not safe for me to be slim and attractive..."

"Even though my (husband/wife/best friend, etc.) tries to sabotage my weight-loss efforts..."

"Even though my (mother/father, etc.) criticizes me whenever I start to lose weight..."

"Even though I won't be able to blame my problems on being overweight if I am thin..."

"Even though I've been overweight for so long, I don't know who I'll be, or how I'll act when I become thinner..."

Self-Sabotage

If you don't know where your resistance is coming from, try answering the following questions:

What are the pluses of maintaining your current weight?

"Even though I'm familiar and comfortable with the overweight me..."

"Even though I feel safer when I weigh more..."

What are the pluses of maintaining your eating habits?

"Even though it is so much easier to eat whatever I want..."

"Even though I need my comfort food..."

Then ask these questions:

What are the minuses of losing weight?

"Even though I can't hide behind my weight..."

"Even though it's so much work to lose weight…"

"Even though I don't want men/women to pay attention to me…"

What are the minuses of changing your eating habits?

"Even though I can't use food to avoid uncomfortable feelings…"

"Even though I need the distraction of overeating and hating myself…"

Spend some time with these questions. Grab pen and paper, or a computer, and write whatever comes to mind. Don't censor or judge. Just write. See what comes up. Be prepared for surprises.

Flow Tapping and Aspects

During or after a round of tapping, the intensity of the original emotion you were working with may decrease. As this happens, it is very possible that other feelings will emerge. These are the different "aspects" of an issue mentioned in Chapter Seven. They are simply different parts or layers of the presenting issue.

When there are multiple aspects to an issue, it is important to separate them out as distinct entities to be tapped on. By dealing with all its facets, the issue can be completely resolved.

The best way to work with the different aspects that emerge is to "go with the flow." Tune into the strongest, most painful emotion or aspect, and tap on that feeling and the thoughts you have about that issue. As the pain of the original problem begins to soften and dissolve, and other feelings emerge, new Set-Up statements will suggest themselves.

Continue to tap on whatever feelings and thoughts come up until a resolution has been reached, or you feel that it is time to stop.

Below is a case study that illustrates the use of flow tapping and working with the various aspects of an issue that can arise. Although it is not weight-loss related, it is a good example of how to work with aspects as they arise.

The Stolen Laptops

A woman I'll call Susan was extremely upset because her house had recently been broken into and two laptops had been stolen. She felt angry and violated.

"Even though I am furious because they came into my house and took my computers..."

"Even though I feel so violated..."

As her anger receded, feelings of fear arose.

"Even though I'm afraid that someone could break into our house again and take our things..."

"Even though I feel so vulnerable..."

At this point Susan started to cry. Her feelings of fear actually increased. She realized that what really terrified her was the idea that her two-month old infant, sleeping in the room next to hers, could have been hurt.

"Even though I'm so upset that the robber(s) could have hurt my daughter...."

"Even though I am petrified that someone might break into our house again and harm her..."

"Even though I am so scared...How can we protect her?..."

"Even though I love her more than my own life and I feel helpless to protect her..."

As Susan tapped, her fear abated. In this calmer state she realized that she could protect her family and her home by installing an adequate security system, and vowed to do so as soon as she got home. The solution occurred to her once she had neutralized her fear and felt calm and in control.

Limiting Beliefs

Limiting beliefs may be another block to success. You could harbor many negative ideas about your ability to lose weight and/or to keep the weight off once you've reached your goal. You may also have doubts that EFT or hypnosis can work. EFT can neutralize negative thoughts and beliefs, just as it defuses negative emotions.

Beliefs are held in place by their emotional investment. When you have a limiting belief and you use EFT, it drains the negative emotion away from the limiting belief, weakening the strength of that belief. Positive beliefs will then emerge and take the place of the negative belief.

Here are some negative beliefs you may be harboring.

"I can't lose weight because no one in my family is thin, or can get thin."

"I don't believe I can change."

"I can't handle my life without my favorite comfort foods."
"It's not safe to be thin."

"EFT won't work; it's just too weird."

"Hypnosis may work for other people, but not for me."

If you identify with any of these statements, choose one that strongly resonates with you. Using the SUD rating, notice on a scale of zero to ten how true a particular statement is for you. Ten is very true, and zero is not true at all. Now begin to tap, putting "Even though" in front of the negative statement you've chosen, and "I deeply and completely accept myself" at the end.

"Even though I can't reach my weight loss goal, I deeply and completely accept myself."

"Even though I can't maintain my ideal weight for long…"

"Even though I can't lose weight because no one in my family is thin, or can get thin…"

"Even though I don't believe I can change…"

"Even though I can't handle my life without my favorite comfort foods…"

"Even though it's not safe for me to be thin…"

"Even though I don't think EFT will work; it's just too weird…

"Even though hypnosis may work for other people, I don't think it will work for me, and…"

Check in again to access the subjective truth of the statement you are tapping on. On a scale of zero to ten, how true does the statement feel to you now? Continue tapping until the number you identify has been reduced to a two or below.

Self-Acceptance

Nothing will bring your weight-loss progress to a screeching halt faster than self-loathing. It creates a knot in the energy system that can only be untangled with a healthy dose of compassion, forgiveness, and the consistent application of EFT.

You may have been wondering why the EFT set-up phrase includes the affirmation "I deeply and completely accept myself." It is there to remove the negative emotions directed toward the self. Energy will not flow smoothly as long as you are tying yourself up in knots energetically with feelings of blame and self-loathing.

It is just about impossible to lose weight and keep it off if you are constantly criticizing yourself. If you frequently berate yourself for being "bad" when you make poor food choices, if you suffer feelings of disgust when you see your image in the mirror, if you beat yourself up for regaining weight, then permanent weight loss will be elusive.

The default Set-Up phrase "I deeply and completely accept myself" paves the way for healing by shifting the locked-up energy of self-abasement using the softer energy of self-acceptance.

You might wish to try some of these variations of the self-acceptance phrase:

> *"Even though I feel angry with myself for not losing weight, I deeply and completely accept myself with kindness and compassion."*

> *"Even though I am disgusted with my behavior around food, I totally accept myself without judgment. I acknowledge how difficult this is for me."*

You may find it difficult to believe that you can or should accept yourself. Keep using the acceptance phrase anyway. You might wish to alter it slightly to reflect your self-doubt. Here are a few examples:

"Even though I can't yet accept myself, I can and do acknowledge myself and my efforts."

"Even though I can't quite accept myself, I'll be OK."

"Even though I can't yet fully and completely accept myself, I am willing to accept the possibility that I will accept myself in the future."

Maybe you are worried that if you accept yourself, it means you are accepting your behavior, and if you do, nothing will change; you'll return to your old eating patterns and the weight will pile back on. This is not true. You are simply stating that you accept yourself despite your flaws, your struggles, and your very human frailties.

And remember that if self-loathing were actually helpful, you'd be stick-thin by now.

A Self-Acceptance Practice
If you're constantly focused on your faults and have trouble seeing the good in yourself, give this practice a try.

At the end of the day, write down three to five positive things you did. They don't have to be huge efforts. Small, everyday, from-the-heart stuff will work quite well. Then tap as follows:

"Even though I think I am (no good, weak, a failure, etc.), I choose to remember that today I (made someone smile, took care of my children, cooked a great dinner, etc.)."

Do this every night for at least two weeks. If you do it often enough, you will be able to call up the hundreds of ways that you make this world a better place. Continue until you're convinced

that you really are innately wonderful. Try to give yourself uncon-
ditional love and kindness. It is part of the healing process.

The Choices Method

As stated previously, the default set-up phrase "I deeply and
completely accept myself" is a very powerful and effective antidote for the self-criticism and self-judgment so prevalent among
those struggling with weight and food issues. However, when the
intensity of your feelings or negative beliefs has decreased to a
three or lower, it can be very useful to inject affirmations in place
of the default love and acceptance phrase. The effectiveness of
affirmations increases when combined with the power of EFT.

The EFT Choices Method, developed by Dr. Patricia Carrington,
is a variation of the default Set-Up Phrase "I deeply and completely accept myself." With her method, you replace the self-
acceptance affirmation in the Set-Up with a Choice statement that
addresses your targeted problem. This affirmation is the opposite
of the negative statement contained in the first portion of the Set-
Up Phrase.

This Choice statement is an expression of what you truly desire. It
expresses the outcome that you wish to create.

This is how the method works:

Create your Set-Up Phrase:
1. Identify the negative cognition (thought, attitude, feel-
    ing) you want to eliminate.

2. Estimate your level of intensity about this problem, on
    the 0–10 SUD scale.

3. Formulate a choice that is roughly the opposite of the
    negative thought; an antidote to it. For example, "*I
    choose to feel confident in my ability to lose weight*" would be

an opposite choice for the negative belief *"I don't think I can reach my weight-loss goal."*

4. Combine the negative thought with the positive choice to create a Choices Set-Up. For example, *"Even though I don't think I can reach my weight-loss goal, I choose to feel confident in my ability to lose weight."*

5. Tap the Karate Chop spot three times while repeating your Choices Set-Up Phrase.

Next you will tap three separate rounds. You will state the negative phrase in the first round, the positive in the second, and then alternate the negative and positive phrases during the third.

First round
Do one complete round of EFT using the negative thought as the reminder phrase. Repeat *"I can't reach my weight-loss goal"* at each tapping point.

Second round
Follow immediately with another complete round of EFT, using the positive choice as a reminder phrase. Repeat *"I choose to feel confident in my ability to lose weight"* at each tapping point.

Third round
Perform a third round of EFT, alternating the negative thought and positive choice as you move between tapping points:

1. At the first tapping point (eyebrow), use the negative statement for the reminder phrase: *"I can't reach my weight-loss goal."*

2. At the next tapping point (side of eye), use the positive choice as the reminder phrase: *"I choose to feel confident in my ability to lose weight."*

3. At the next tapping point (under the eye), again use the negative statement for the reminder phrase.

4. Continue alternating the negative and positive until you have tapped all of the EFT points, ending with the positive choice at the Top of the Head point.

It is important that, on the third round, you always start with the negative statement and end with the positive.

When you've finished the three rounds, estimate your new SUD level. Repeat the choices trio until you get your SUD level down to two or below.

Here are some examples of choice statements.

"Even though losing weight is just too hard, I choose to let it be easy."

"Even though I feel stressed out and want to eat, I choose to feel calm and at ease."

"Even though I feel guilty for eating _____, I choose to forgive myself and commit to making better food choices in the future."

Some people never incorporate the Choices Method into their EFT practice and still get great results. Others find that it enhances their results exponentially. Experiment with it and decide for yourself.

To learn more about the Choices Method, refer to Dr. Carrington's website: *www.masteringeft.com.*

CALL TO ACTION

1. Be aware of resistance to the weight-loss process. Examine negative beliefs about your ability to lose weight, as well as any other negative and judgmental thoughts. Use EFT to dissolve resistance and neutralize negativity and self-criticism.

2. Practice developing positive Choice statements.

3. Continue to practice mindfulness, paying close attention to your feelings and to the eating process itself. Apply EFT when appropriate.

4. Continue to listen daily to the hypnosis recording, "Freedom from Excess Weight." or to the recording of your choice. (See Appendix.)

Chapter Nine
HEALING YOUR PAST

If your weight loss is progressing smoothly and steadily, you may not require the information presented in this chapter. You need only continue paying attention to what and why you eat, work with any resistance that arises, and continue daily practice of EFT and hypnosis.

If, however, you find yourself repeatedly slipping back into old eating habits despite your best efforts, your eating patterns might stem from a difficult and painful past. Your relationship to food could have developed as a way to cope with neglect, family dysfunction, and/or abuse. If this is true for you, it may be helpful to engage in the task of exploring and healing your past.

Signals that Healing Past Memories May be Beneficial

You may need to do this kind of exploration if any of the following patterns emerge:

- Painful memories frequently surface when you tap for current feelings or problems.
- The same uncomfortable emotions, such as anger or sadness, emerge repeatedly when you explore present emotional issues that trigger overeating.
- You successfully neutralize all of your food cravings, but find painful feelings such as anger or sadness arising when you stop overeating.
- Weight loss stalls, despite your regular use of EFT and hypnosis.
- You have been struggling with your weight or struggling with food issues since you were young.

Overview

Thus far you have been using EFT primarily to neutralize cravings and the emotional discomfort that prompt overeating, and to alter the negative beliefs that have sabotaged your weight-loss progress in the past. You did this by focusing on an uncomfortable emotional or physical feeling, or a negative belief, and tapping on that identified feeling or belief.

Using EFT to heal past experiences that contribute to your present eating habits is a bit more complex. It requires a certain amount of detective work to uncover the events, the *core issues* that initially triggered your tendency to overeat. And the tapping techniques you will use are more lengthy and multifaceted.

How EFT Heals
As previously stated, EFT rests upon the following theory:

"The cause of all negative emotions is a disruption in the energy system."

Thus painful experiences of the past that elicited negative emotions—such as shame and self-criticism—created a disruption in the energy system. These disruptions can be eliminated by the targeted use of EFT. EFT can eradicate the emotional impact of these events. You will retain the memory, but not the painful feelings they caused. The emotional charge will be neutralized.

Discovering the Core

The Present
To get to the bottom of what makes you overeat, begin by asking questions about recent experiences. Think about an incident that precipitated overeating.
- What was happening at the time?
- Who were you with?

- How did you feel?
- When in the past did you feel the same way?

Alternatively, instead of focusing on one incident, you can identify recurring feelings that trigger overeating. For instance, feelings of anger, irritation, or anxiety may often precipitate the urge to eat. Fill in the blank:

"When I feel _____, I want to eat."

"This _____ feeling makes me want to eat _____."

When in the past did you feel this way? What event or events prompted these same emotions?

The Past

You can also begin by examining your past instead of the present.
- What traumas occurred in your past? Are you using food to numb the pain from this incident(s) or stuff it down?
- What losses from the past trigger overeating?

You can look at the role food played when you were a child.
- What attitudes about food did you learn or develop? Did you learn to associate eating with celebrations? Tragedies? Were you given food when you needed comforting?
- When did you first overeat and why? When did you first turn to food for comfort, distraction, etc.?

If you're still having trouble finding a core issue:
- Guess! If there were a deeper emotion underlying this problem, what might it be?
- Ask yourself, if you could live your life over again, what person or event would you prefer to skip?

The EFT Healing Process

Once you have identified a core issue, there are several EFT techniques that can be used to neutralize it. You won't have to apply EFT to every painful memory. Usually moving through six or seven incidents related to an issue will be enough to heal it.

For instance, if the primary feeling that fuels overeating is a sense of shame because you were often criticized as a child, choose five or six of your most painful memories of being criticized and apply EFT to each one.

One of the most remarkable characteristics of EFT is its ability to heal the energetic disruption caused by an upsetting event, thereby neutralizing the painful feelings elicited by the event. The event becomes simply something unfortunate that happened to you. The issue is resolved and the incident can be recalled without any emotional response.

The Importance of Being Specific

Often general themes will present themselves. For example, "My father always criticized me" is a broad statement that might reflect your father's behavior toward you throughout your childhood. If you tap on this statement, however, you won't get very far. EFT will be much more effective when applied to specific times when you were criticized.

You won't have to tap on every related memory, just a few. Tapping through and healing several events will create a generalized effect on the issue as a whole. Think of the broader issue as a tabletop, with the legs representing specific events from the past that contribute to the current problem. By collapsing some or all of the legs, the tabletop will become unstable and fall over, providing emotional relief from the bigger issue.

Aspects

Aspects, as you recall, are different facets of an issue that may contribute to your emotional distress. While some painful experiences have only one primary aspect, others might have several. After you tap on one feeling, another one may emerge. If this happens, tap on the newer feeling, bringing it down to a two or lower on the SUD scale. Continue with this process until all the aspects are cleared.

Healing Techniques

Two of the most powerful and effective methods for neutralizing painful memories are the Story Technique and the Movie Technique, described below.

The Story Technique

This method involves narrating a specific event and stopping to tap whenever you get to the emotionally intense parts of it. Each of the stopping points represents another aspect of the issue that may take you to even deeper issues.

Here are the steps to the process:

1. Begin to relate the story at a point before the painful part of the story took place. An example might be having lunch with a friend just before being involved in a car accident.

2. Stop recounting the story as soon as you feel any emotional intensity surface and tap until that feeling has been neutralized. Then continue telling the story.

3. When you've recounted the whole story, repeat the process, looking for any remaining distress, and clearing that discomfort with EFT as you proceed. Do this until you can tell the story without emotional discomfort.

4. Finally, close your eyes and imagine the whole event as vividly as possible. Try to get yourself upset by exaggerating the sights, sounds, and feelings associated with it. If there is any emotional charge left, you will have uncovered an important aspect or underlying cause. Use EFT for whatever comes up, until you cannot get upset about the issue by imagining it or talking about it.

The Movie Technique

Here are the guidelines for another method useful for healing the past, known as the Movie Technique.

1. Identify a painful or traumatic incident from your past. Ask yourself, *"If this event were a movie, how long would it last?"* Ideally it should only be two to three minutes long.

2. Give the event a title.

3. Run the movie in your mind and evaluate the intensity of feeling on a scale of zero to 10. If you can't come up with a number, just guess.

4. Next, do several rounds of EFT on *"this* _____ *movie."* At the end of each round, check out the zero to 10 intensity scale and continue to apply EFT if necessary.

5. Go through the movie in your mind, starting with a low-intensity segment, but stop and tap whenever you feel any emotional intensity.

6. Then, mentally run through the movie again, from beginning to end, tapping on intense aspects as they come up, until the movie no longer has a charge to it.

7. Finally, when the intensity seems to be resolved, go through the movie one last time, but exaggerate the sights, sounds, colors, etc., and consciously try to get upset about

it. If you find more pockets of intensity, keep repeating the steps above until they are gone. When you can no longer get upset, your work is done.

Case Studies

These case studies are excerpts from actual sessions with former clients. Their names, of course, have been changed. The sessions provide illustrations of both the Movie and Story Techniques. They offer examples of how to work with aspects and emphasize the importance of being specific. They also demonstrate the flowing nature of an EFT session.

Jenny

In trying to discover the root cause of Jenny's overeating, I asked her to tell me what was going on the last time she binged. She recounted a conversation she had had with her oldest daughter. Jenny felt angry because her daughter was speaking in derogatory tones about her own daughter, Jenny's granddaughter. Jenny knew that her granddaughter was not getting the attention she needed or deserved, and that she was being criticized unjustly. We began tapping, using these set-up statements:

"Even though I am so angry at my daughter for the terrible way she treats my granddaughter..."

"Even though I am mad because she is too critical..."

Her anger gave way to sadness.

"Even though I feel so sad when I think about the way my granddaughter is being treated..."

"Even though it hurts me to think of my granddaughter being criticized and misunderstood because I know how that feels..."

Jenny then spontaneously remembered incidents from her own childhood when her mother was not present for her, did not give her the care or attention she needed, and was callous and insensitive to Jenny's needs. These experiences were the source of the deep pain she was assuaging with food.

I asked Jenny to think of an incident, the first one that came to mind, in which her mother had been insensitive and hurtful. I suggested she imagine this event as a short movie and give it a title. She named this "movie" *My First Period*. When I asked what she felt as she imagined the movie and asked her to rate her emotional intensity, she replied that she felt angry, and her intensity level was a strong 10.

I had Jenny tap, using the following Set-Up statement:

"Even though I am so angry about My First Period*…"*

When her anger subsided to a five, I asked her to tell me about her "movie."

Jenny was 11 years old when she began menstruating. Her mother had not informed her about the menstrual cycle, and Jenny was alarmed and frightened when she unexpectedly found herself bleeding profusely. As she recounted this incident, her anger once again escalated.

"Even though I am so angry at my mother for not telling me about my period…"

"Even though I can't believe she didn't tell me about something so important…"

When the intensity of her anger came down to a two, Jenny continued her story.

When she called her mother to tell her what had happened and to ask why and what she should do, her mother laughed with derision. She told her daughter it was no big deal. As Jenny recounted these events, she again felt intense anger, so we tapped.

"Even though I feel so angry that she laughed at me...I was just a little girl, and I was frightened..."

"Even though I am so mad at her; she was so insensitive..."

Anger turned to sadness, and a deep sense of grief washed over Jenny as she recalled her feelings of shame and abandonment.

"Even though I feel so sad, I really needed my mother to comfort me and explain what was going on..."

"Even though she made me feel something was wrong with me for not knowing what was going on..."

"Even though she made fun of me for being so upset..."

As Jenny's shame and sadness decreased, a sense of calmness and equanimity returned to her. When I asked her to think about the incident again and to tell me if any emotional pain remained, she said there was none. I had her tell me the whole story once more to make sure every aspect had been neutralized. As she did so, she recalled something else her mother had said, and a sense of hurt arose once more.

"Even though my mother said I was making a big deal out of nothing..."

"Even though she made fun of me because I was crying..."

After we tapped down her distress, and calmness returned once more, I asked Jenny to describe the incident again to make sure we had completely neutralized the pain of the memory. I repeated phrases her mother had used, mimicking her mother's tone of voice in an effort to elicit any remaining hurt she might still harbor. When I got no reaction from her, I knew we had healed that particular incident.

We continued, over the course of several sessions, to tap on various memories that brought up feelings of anger, sadness, and shame. When we had resolved five or six of these, Jenny's binge eating began to dissipate. She felt calmer, less anxious, and less driven to overeat. She began to lose weight.

More importantly, Jenny felt happier and more at peace. We continued to use EFT for forgiveness, and she gradually released the anger and resentment that she had carried inside for so long.

Donna

Donna was a member of one of my weight-loss groups. She was diligent in her practice of EFT for food cravings, and she listened to her hypnosis CD every day. In the first few weeks of the 10-week program, she came to each session with a big smile on her face, excited and happy to be losing weight with relative ease.

One evening about halfway through the program, however, Donna came to the group looking absolutely miserable. When I asked her what was wrong, she said that she was struggling once again with binge eating.

When queried about the previous week, she told me that she had been thinking a lot about her father, who had been dead for about six years. He had been critical and insensitive toward her as a child and young adult, and she felt intense anger toward him.

Donna had been using food to deal with the feelings of hurt and anger she had toward her father. When she stopped overeating, all the feelings she had been stuffing down began to surface.

I asked her to recount an incident that illustrated her conflicts with her father and to tell it as if it were a story.

Donna wanted very much to take ballet lessons when she was a young girl, and when she was in the fourth grade, her father finally acquiesced. However, the day she was to begin, she had to stay after school for reading a storybook during geography class. (She loved to read and found it difficult to focus on subjects she was not interested in.) When her father came to fetch her, her fourth grade teacher told him why Donna was being disciplined.

As she recalled the image of two large adults towering over her, waves of shame washed over her.

"Even though I felt so ashamed..."

"Even though I was so embarrassed..."

They shook their heads and talked about what a bad little girl she was for not paying attention in class.

"Even though they made me cry..."
"Even though they seemed glad that I was crying..."

"Even though I'm so angry when I think about that because I was just a little girl..."

When Donna and her father finally left school, he told her that she certainly could not take dancing lessons after that. Donna was heartbroken.

"Even though I was so sad and disappointed that I couldn't take ballet lessons..."

"Even though I felt really mad, because I had already been punished enough..."

Donna and I engaged in several private sessions after this, exploring similar memories that aroused hurt and anger. Gradually those feelings abated and her weight loss resumed.

Sharon

Sharon was a kind and friendly woman who had struggled with food for most of her life. She seemed like a happy person, laughing easily and often. But sadness was very close to the surface, and whenever we began tapping, tears would immediately start welling in her eyes.

Sharon had been taught that it was not okay to look sad, and had been criticized for "making that face." We did some tapping on several incidents when she was criticized for crying or looking unhappy.

I then asked Sharon about her earliest memories of overeating. She recalled her grandmother's funeral when she was age six. That was when she learned to associate eating with sadness. Eating was an acceptable way to share grief and loss, and it made her feel better.

As she began to retell this event, she felt overwhelmingly sad.

"Even though I feel so sad..."

"Even though I felt such loss..."

"Even though I miss her still..."

Sharon noticed an ache in her stomach. I asked her to describe the pain and note its intensity.

"Even though I have this tight, dark ache in my belly..."

We tapped on this, and the bellyache decreased. However, she then noticed a constricted feeling in her chest. We then "chased the pain" by tapping on the next physical symptom that presented itself.

"Even though I have this knot in my chest and I can't take a deep breath..."

The tightness in her chest dissolved and she could breathe deeply once again, but noticed her throat now felt tight.

"Even though my throat feels tight, as if I have swallowed something without chewing it well enough..."

We tapped until her throat felt normal once again.

When we checked in with her feelings about her grandmother's passing, her sadness was gone, and she felt at peace.

Over the course of several sessions, we tapped on other events in which she was not allowed to express sadness, often moving back and forth between physical and emotional discomfort. We also used EFT to change her beliefs about sadness and eating.

"Even though it's not okay to look sad..."

"Even though it's okay to eat when I'm sad..."

The deep sadness buried beneath her happy façade began to dissipate, as did her need to eat compulsively.

The Personal Peace Procedure

Another method for healing the past is the more general approach of Gary Craig's "Personal Peace Procedure." You can use it to alleviate any and all pain associated with your past, whether it has directly contributed to your current eating issues or not. It involves making a list of every bothersome event from your past and using EFT to dissolve the pain associated with that event.

Here are the instructions:

1. Make a list of every painful event you can remember. We have all lived through many difficult moments. Make a list of between 30 and 50 of yours. This list may evolve over a period of time.

2. Give each specific event a title as though it were a mini-movie. Examples: *My father called me stupid; My brother hit me hard; I almost drowned.*

3. When the list is complete, pick out the most painful events and apply EFT to each of them until you no longer get upset when you think about them. Be sure to notice any aspects that may come up and apply EFT to them accordingly. Tap on each aspect until it is resolved.

4. If you cannot get in touch with your feelings about an event, apply 10 full rounds of EFT on it from every angle you can think of. After you have tapped on the most painful memories, move on to the others on your list.

5. Apply EFT to one event per day for three months. Then notice how much better you feel, both emotionally and physically. Note, too, how much calmer you feel. Observe the improvement in your relationships.

Even though you have not focused on incidents specifically related to food, in this process you may notice an overall decrease in your struggles with food. As discussed previously, many food issues have their origins in early childhood distress.

Gary Craig's EFT Manual

Although EFT is a very simple technique, there is an art to it. To plumb the depth of your emotional issues, you will have to become skilled in this art. Proficiency will develop with knowledge and practice. Gary Craig's "The EFT Manual" will supply you with the former. Practice and experience will provide the latter.

Getting Professional Help

The work of exploring and healing your past can be very difficult. If you discover a lot of pain and heartache as you engage in this process, get professional help. A qualified therapist will be especially helpful if this is the first time you have examined these issues. And if you have suffered childhood abuse of any kind—physical, emotional and/or sexual—then professional support from a qualified therapist is imperative.

You may feel hesitant about engaging in this deeper work, especially if you think that dredging up the past will only bring pain. But healing *is* possible. And working with an EFT-trained psychotherapist can accelerate the process while minimizing the emotional distress.

CALL TO ACTION:

1. If appropriate, begin the work of digging deeper and healing your past. Get help from a professional therapist and/or EFT practitioner if this process feels too difficult or overwhelming.

2. Explore the Personal Peace Procedure

3. Continue to practice mindfulness, paying close attention to your feelings and to the eating process itself. Apply EFT when appropriate.

4. Continue to listen daily to the hypnosis recording, "Freedom from Excess Weight." or to the recording of your choice. (See Appendix.)

Chapter Ten
THE STRESS/WEIGHT CONNECTION

Stress can make you fat. It can increase your appetite, your cravings for refined carbohydrates, your blood sugar and your insulin levels. It can decrease your metabolism and your ability to make healthy food choices. In short, excess stress is capable of bringing your weight-loss progress to a screeching halt.

This is a challenging issue. Life can be hectic and demanding. However, you can develop the ability to stay centered and composed in the course of a challenging day. And you can do this without turning to food. With practice, insight, and a willingness to take care of yourself, you can change your response to the pressures and concerns of the day without derailing your weight-loss efforts.

What is Stress?
Stress is the emotional and physical strain caused by your response to pressure. While a certain amount of tension keeps you alert and challenged, too much can harm your health, your relationships, and your enjoyment of life. It can also make the commitment to your exercise and food plan next to impossible to maintain.

Stress overload erupts when you find that you are required to handle too much; too much work, too much responsibility, too much pressure. Life becomes overly demanding, and you may feel anxious, tense, frustrated, and overwhelmed.

Common physical reactions to stress overload include tension, anxiety, irritability, insomnia, and an inability to concentrate. Feelings of helplessness and hopelessness are also common. Physical symptoms can include headache, stomach upset, tight muscles, difficulty breathing, and fatigue.

Food cravings are another response to stress. Food can feel like a soothing and dependable friend, easing your anxiety and providing immediate comfort. The relief it provides, though, is short-lived, while resulting weight problems from overeating are not.

What Causes Stress?
The potential causes of stress are numerous and highly individual. What you consider stressful depends on many factors, including your personality, general outlook on life, problem-solving abilities, and social support system. Something that's stressful to you may not faze someone else; they may even find that particular stimulus energizing and enjoyable.

Although you can't always change your circumstances, you can learn to control your *response* to those situations. In addition, you can develop techniques that will reduce the effects of stress on your mental and physical health.

How Stress Makes You Fat

Stress promotes weight gain in several ways. Both physical and emotional factors contribute to the tendency to eat more and move less. And a number of physiological responses are initiated which make losing weight extremely difficult.

The Time Crunch
Stress is often due to feelings of pressure and overwhelm. You may feel that there is too much to do and not enough time to do it in. If you are feeling overwhelmed by all of the demands placed upon you, you will find it extremely difficult to make exercise and eating healthfully a priority.

Comfort Foods
Overeating is a common response to stress. When you are immersed in feelings of anxiety or apprehension, turning to food,

particularly unhealthy carbohydrates such as candy and chips, is a common response because ingesting these tasty junk foods can soothe and comfort you.

As explained in Chapter Five, refined carbohydrates can boost the production of the neurotransmitters serotonin and beta-endorphin. A rise in serotonin levels creates a sense of calmness, focus, optimism, and control. An increase in beta-endorphins may ease emotional distress, producing a sense of well-being.

Your physiological response to stress, however, is not just due to an unconscious desire for these feel-good brain chemicals. Stress can also increase your appetite via a biomechanical response known as the *fight or flight response*.

The Fight or Flight Response

The drive to eat when you are stressed out is physical as well as emotional, a result of the hard-wired reaction to stress known as the fight or flight response (also known as the *stress response*). This is a series of biochemical changes that prepares you to deal with threats or danger.

Any problem, imagined or real, will cause the cerebral cortex to send an alarm to the hypothalamus. The hypothalamus then stimulates the sympathetic nervous system to make a series of changes in the body. Your heart rate, breathing rate, muscle tension, metabolism, and blood pressure all increase. Your hands and feet get cold as blood is directed away from your extremities and digestive system into the larger muscles that can help you fight or run. Your adrenaline glands start to secrete corticoids, which inhibit digestion, reproduction, growth, tissue repair, and the responses of your immune and inflammatory systems.

Once the perceived danger has passed, the body must replenish the energy it lost while engaged in the stress response. It accomplishes this through eating and rest. The body then resumes its normal mode of functioning until the next time the stress response is triggered.

This primitive stress response developed out of a need to fight or flee from a life-threatening event such as being chased by a wild animal. However, today you are much more likely to experience a kind of chronic, low-grade stress that occurs when a number of crises follow one another, or when a lot of little stressors accumulate. As long as feelings of tension persist, you remain wound up and ready for action. And hungry.

Cortisol

Cortisol is a one of the primary hormones secreted by the body during times of stress. High cortisol levels prompt an increase in appetite. This was a helpful response when stress was a short-lived event that required doing battle or running away. Such activities required using up large stores of energy that would later be replaced.

The type of stress you face today, however, is rarely life-threatening. It doesn't usually require a sudden physical response, nor does it peak and then diminish. You are much more likely to suffer from a constant, low-level tension that remains with you throughout the day. As a result, cortisol levels often remain chronically high, along with increased hunger.

What kind of foods do you crave when you're feeling anxious or frustrated and cortisol levels are running high? Starchy carbohydrates, of course! You crave cookies, candy, bread; in short, anything that will raise your blood-sugar levels quickly and give you the boost of energy your body is looking for.

In addition to increasing your appetite, cortisol contributes to weight gain in several other ways. It causes a decline in muscle mass, lowers metabolism, increases blood-sugar levels, and decreases insulin sensitivity. What's more, elevated cortisol levels will cause stress-induced weight gain to land primarily in the abdominal area. This is the unhealthiest place to carry excess weight, because it puts you at risk for heart disease, diabetes, and certain types of cancer.

Chronically high cortisol levels can also adversely affect your health in a number of other ways. They can

- Impair your immune response, increasing your risk of infection, inflammatory and autoimmune conditions, and possibly cancer
- Increase the likelihood of depression, anxiety, shifting moods of anger and frustration, memory and learning impairment
- Cause or aggravate insomnia
- Increase your risk of heart attack
- Cause reproductive dysfunction, including irregular menstrual cycles and decreased fertility; increase premenstrual syndrome (PMS), risk of postpartum depression, and discomfort during menopause and perimenopause

Sleep Deprivation
Lack of sleep is both a stressor and a response to stress. Feeling overwhelmed and pressured can make getting to sleep or finding enough time to sleep difficult.

Sleep, or lack of it, affects the body in many ways:

- Lack of sleep is a stressor. As mentioned before, it increases the production of cortisol, a major hormone that increases appetite and abdominal fat. High levels of cortisol can trigger insomnia, creating a vicious cycle.
- The absence of deep, restorative sleep prevents the body from creating a reserve of serotonin, which leads to food cravings and overeating (as well as depression).
- Without enough recuperative sleep, your pituitary gland will not produce significant amounts of growth hormone (rhGH), which assists in the building of muscle and the

loss of fat. Without sufficient levels of this hormone, you may lose muscle (slowing down your metabolism), store the food you eat as fat instead of burning it for energy, and retain excess weight.

- Lack of sleep can trigger food cravings and overeating as your body attempts to fuel up due to low energy. And self-control can be very difficult when you are tired.

Sleep Apnea

Obstructive sleep apnea occurs when breathing is blocked during sleep. People who have this condition usually snore after falling asleep. (Not all snorers have sleep apnea, however, most people with sleep apnea snore.) Once they're asleep, their snoring gets louder and louder. Then it suddenly stops, because their throat tissue has relaxed to the point at which it is blocking their upper airway. They then snort or gasp, and breathing is restored.

Since the person with sleep apnea does not usually wake up during the process, they are often unaware that they have repeatedly stopped breathing. As one might expect, people with undiagnosed sleep apnea often feel exhausted during the day without knowing why. They also tend to wake up with headaches, feel "foggy-brained," and are at risk for falling asleep at inappropriate times, such as while driving. In addition, sleep apnea can cause high blood pressure. When the brain is deprived of oxygen, the heart has to work harder to restore adequate blood flow.

Although thin people suffer from obstructive sleep apnea, excess weight can make you more likely to develop this common sleep disorder. The result is a vicious cycle—for the reasons described above, not getting enough sleep makes it harder to lose weight, which in turn makes one more likely to develop sleep apnea.

There are several ways to treat the disorder, the most common of which is the use of a device called a CPAP (Continuous Positive Airway Pressure). If you suspect that you have sleep apnea, talk to your doctor about setting up a sleep study. While it's easy to dismiss the significance of having sleep apnea, proper diagnosis and treatment can change your life. It may also help you lose weight.

Solutions to Stress-Driven Overeating

So what can you do about the perpetual stress that is not only making your life difficult, but putting you at risk for obesity and all of the other physical and mental health problems that can accompany it?

The best approach is to learn stress management and coping skills. There are many effective techniques available.

In this chapter the following methods will be explored:
- Developing stress resilience with daily *relaxation practices* that elicit the relaxation response. There are a variety of techniques you can use, including meditation, progressive relaxation, guided imagery, and affirmations.
- Dealing with stress in the moment by using *deep breathing* and *EFT*
- Making appropriate *lifestyle choices* that will reduce your physical and emotional response to stress. These include eating well, exercising consistently, getting enough sleep, becoming more mindful, and nourishing your spirit.

The Relaxation Response

During the late 1960's, the president of the Mind/Body Medical Institute, Herbert Benson, M.D., studied meditation and found that it produced a splendid counterbalancing mechanism to the fight-or-flight response. He named this mechanism the Relaxation Response.

The Relaxation Response is a state of deep rest that reverses the physical and emotional responses to stress: it decreases heart rate, blood pressure, and muscle tension, slows and deepens the breath, and relaxes formally tight muscles. If practiced regularly, it can have lasting effects on the way you respond to stress throughout the day, and can improve your health.

Several types of meditation were described in Chapter Seven. In addition to helping you to become more mindful, these techniques will also trigger the Relaxation Response. There are also a number of other ways to elicit the Relaxation Response. Let's look at a few.

Progressive Relaxation

In a progressive relaxation practice, you simply relax every muscle, one by one. You can start at the toes and work your way up to your head. Or you can start at the crown of your head and move downward. Here is a short, progressive relaxation script.

> *Sit or lie down, and get comfortable.*
> *Begin by taking a few deep, relaxing breaths, in and out.*
> *Allow the muscles of your forehead to relax.*
> *Relax the muscles around your eyes, cheeks, and mouth.*
> *Allow the jaw to relax and slacken.*
> *Allow the muscles of your stomach to relax, and your lower back.*
> *Relax your hips, your buttocks.*
> *Relax your thighs, your calves, and shins.*
> *Relax your feet and your toes.*
> *Relax your neck, and let your shoulders sink downward.*
> *Relax your upper back and your chest.*
> *Relax your upper arms, your lower arms, your hands.*
> *Relax each and every finger.*
> *Now scan your body to see if there is any tension left.*
> *If there is, just breathe into that tightness and let it go.*
> *Enjoy this sense of deep, peaceful relaxation.*

Guided Imagery

Guided imagery is a method of using your imagination to bring you into a relaxed, focused state. Using all of your senses, your body will respond as though what you are imagining were real.

To test this, imagine a lemon in great detail: the smell, the color, the texture of the peel. As you continue to imagine the lemon, imagine taking a bite of it. Feel the juice squirting into your mouth and experience the sour taste. Many people salivate when they do this. This exercise demonstrates how your body can respond to what you are imagining.

The *special-place guided imagery* described below involves envisioning a place where you feel comfortable, safe, relaxed, and at ease. The idea is to imagine this place with all of your senses; the way it feels, looks, sounds, and smells. The more you can enlist your imagination in this exercise, the more helpful and effective it will be.

Sit or lie down, and get comfortable. Perform the progressive relaxation process described above, relaxing yourself from head to toe.

Now imagine yourself in a place where you feel safe and peaceful, at ease, and at home. This might be someplace you've been to before, or someplace you imagine. Just let the image come to you.

Notice your surroundings. What do they look like? What do they feel like? What do you hear? What kind of aromas are you aware of? Making full use of your imagination, employ all of your senses to mentally explore the sights, the sounds, the smells, and the sensations of this place. Immerse yourself in its loveliness and beauty.

As you explore this special place, find a spot that feels particularly good to you. Choose a spot where you feel very calm, centered, and at ease. Let this be your "power spot," a place where you draw from the deep sense of peacefulness you feel here. Enjoy the feeling of healing and restfulness.

Stay there as long as you like. When you are ready, take a few deep breaths, open your eyes, and return to regular consciousness.

Affirmations
Another useful technique is the use of affirmations. These are statements of acceptance and positive intent. They are powerful and positive thoughts and statements that you think, speak, and/or write down in order to bring about the manifestation of your goals and to reprogram any negative thought patterns currently instilled in your mind

Here are some affirmations you might use to help you relax and remain calm in the face of life's daily challenges. They will have the most impact if you have first brought yourself into a relaxed state by using progressive relaxation.

- *I remain calm and clear in all situations.*
- *I take deep, cleansing breaths throughout the day.*
- *If I notice that my muscles are tense and tight, I soften and release them with my awareness and my breathing.*
- *I am becoming more patient with myself and others.*
- *I easily let go of worrying about things that I cannot control.*
- *I can sense a deep, peaceful stillness at my center.*

When you say these positive statements quietly to yourself while you are in a relaxed state, they will sink deeply into the subconscious mind, increasing their effectiveness exponentially.

Anchoring
Anchoring refers to the creation of an association between a feeling and a sensory experience. We form natural associations between feelings and external things every day. For example a smell may instantly transport you back to a particular time, a song may bring back memories of a person long gone, and entering a schoolroom may trigger feelings of fear or happiness. Everyone creates links like these, and you create them whether you intend to or not.

You can use this principle deliberately by bringing yourself into a relaxed state and creating a link between that state of relaxation and an action such as taking a deep breath, holding one or more EFT acupoints, and/or saying the word *peace* or *calm* quietly to yourself. You might use a script such as this:

> *Bring one open hand, palm down, to your chest, touching each collarbone point with your spread hand.*
> *As you breathe deeply and hold these points, say the word PEACE quietly to yourself.*
> *Whenever you feel the need to call up these feelings, you will remember to breathe deeply, touch both collarbone points with one hand, and say the word PEACE.*

Hypnosis

Hypnosis, as you already know, is an extremely relaxing experience. A deeply relaxed state is usually a prerequisite to entering trance. Once the body enters this state, the wall between the conscious and the subconscious becomes more permeable, allowing access to the subconscious mind. In this state we are highly suggestible and positive messages can be implanted.

Hypnosis is actually a conglomeration of methods. A hypnosis session may include all of the aforementioned techniques; progressive relaxation, guided imagery, affirmation, and anchoring. Although all of these techniques will elicit the Relaxation Response when used individually, they are even more powerful when combined.

How to Practice These Techniques

You can either memorize these stress management scripts, or record them and then listen to the recording. Use them in combination or practice them separately.

(You may wish to purchase the hypnosis recording entitled "Calm, Centered, and Serene." It combines the four techniques listed above. You will find it on the products page of my website: *www.tlcweightloss.net/products.php*)

Find a quiet and comfortable place where you will be undisturbed. Give yourself 10 to 20 minutes to enjoy the sensation of deep relaxation. Practicing daily will help you to remain calm and peaceful, and you will find yourself handling life's challenging moments with greater ease.

There are many more stress management techniques worth exploring. The Resource section at the end of the book includes information about books and audio programs you may find useful.

Coping with Stress in the Moment

In addition to daily relaxation practices, it is very useful to be familiar with methods that can reduce your tension as it arises. Deep breathing and EFT are two such methods.

Deep Breathing

When you are anxious or upset, your breathing often becomes restricted, and you unknowingly engage in shallow "chest breathing." When this happens, the diaphragm becomes almost frozen in place. Because it can't fully expand, you are less able to take in enough oxygen-rich air. As a result, your heart rate speeds up and your blood pressure increases.

When you don't get sufficient oxygen exchange, the stress response intensifies, even if the stress in your environment does not. This creates a vicious cycle, since the stress response and its attendant hormones keep you in a state of anxiety. Your diaphragm remains stuck, and so do your feelings of agitation.

The antidote to shallow breathing is conscious and deliberate abdominal breathing. When you engage in deep abdominal breathing, you get superb oxygen exchange, taking in generous amounts of oxygen as you inhale, and completely expelling carbon dioxide as you exhale. This kind of breathing can break the stress cycle and bring you back into balance.

Try this simple exercise. Sit or lie down in a comfortable position. Take a deep, slow breath. Place one hand on your chest and one on your abdomen. Observe how they rise as you inhale and lower as you exhale. Enjoy the sensations of deep abdominal breathing for a few moments. Notice how your sense of relaxation and calmness increases.

Here are a few variations on the deep-breathing process. Use them when you find yourself tense or upset, and let them return you to a state of equilibrium.

Make the shift from chest breathing to deep abdominal breathing. Then try the following:

- Count down from ten to one, taking one complete breath—one inhalation, one exhalation—with each number. When you get to one, see how you feel. If you are feeling better, great! If not, repeat.
- As you inhale, count very slowly from one to four. As you exhale, count slowly back down, from four to one. Thus, as you inhale, you say silently to yourself, "One, two, three, four." As you exhale, you say, "Four, three, two, one." Do this for several breaths, until you feel calm and relaxed.
- Choose one of the methods above as you breathe, but this time, pause for a few seconds after each in-breath. Pause again for a few seconds after each out-breath. Do this for several breaths, or for as long as you wish.

EFT for Stress

EFT is a magnificent stress-reducing technique that is literally at your fingertips. Try any of these Set-Up statements the next time you feel stressed.

"Even though I feel stressed out, I deeply and completely accept myself."

"Even though I feel tired, overwhelmed, overworked, anxious, fearful, and pressured, I choose to feel calm and confident."

"Even though I feel stressed out and I want to eat, I choose to feel calm and at ease."*

Notice any *physical sensations* associated with stress, such as pain, tightness, or an inability to breathe deeply. Tap on them.

"Even though I have a headache..."

"Even though I feel a tightness in my stomach..."

"Even though I can't breathe deeply..."

Touch and Breath

Gently touch or rub each EFT acupoint while breathing deeply. Use the EFT Set-Up statements and Reminder Phrases, or focus on the source of tension as you hold each point and breathe.

Lifestyle

Many factors contributing to stress are not in our control. However, we can choose to take care of ourselves, both physically and emotionally. Eating well, exercising, and getting an adequate

---

*These Set-Up phrases employ the Choices Method described in Chapter Eight.

amount of sleep will make you more stress resilient. Deliberately slowing down and paying attention to both your internal and external environment can help break the hurry-worry cycle. And carving out space for your own interests and creative pursuits will allow you to refuel so that you aren't running on empty.

Nutrition
To summarize:

1. **Make healthy food choices.** Make high-quality food selections. Choose fruits, vegetables, and whole grains. Eat an adequate amount of protein and healthy fat at each meal to keep your blood-sugar levels stable.

2. **Avoid sugar and white flour.** These refined carbohydrates have little or no essential nutrients. They provide a short-term boost of energy, but ultimately lead to irritability, moodiness, and food cravings.

3. **Eat when you are hungry, but not starving.** A drop in blood sugar, especially later in the day when your energy levels are low, will prompt sugar/flour cravings that will be hard to ignore. Low blood sugar combined with intense hunger will also make you irritable. If you know you will be eating on the run, be sure to take healthy meals and snacks with you. Some possibilities are sandwiches, yogurt, fruit, string cheese, nuts, and cut-up veggies.

4. **Eat enough.** Diets that restrict caloric intake put a lot of stress on your system. Sooner or later you may rebel with an out-of-control binge.

5. **Respect your body's biorhythms.** The stress hormones cortisol and adrenaline peak early in the day, making you feel energetic, focused, and alert. By mid-morning, these hormone levels start to decline, and by mid-afternoon you usually feel noticeably tired—both physically and mentally.

To keep yourself moving through a mid-afternoon slump, you might be tempted to prop yourself up with caffeine and sugar. This is especially true if you are trying to move at the same speed that you did earlier in the day.

It is important to recognize and respect your natural biorhythms. Try to accomplish your more demanding tasks earlier in the day. Save your less challenging activities for later on.

Exercise

As explained previously, the fight-or-flight response prepares you for action. Your body becomes revved up and ready to go. Moving your body vigorously completes the stress response cycle. Twenty to thirty minutes of moderate exercise can return you to sanity. Exercise is a tremendous mood elevator and stress reducer. And it is a great way to pick yourself up from a mid-afternoon slump. More on exercise in Chapter Eleven.

Adequate Sleep

Seven or eight hours are enough for most people. As stated previously, the price for sleep deprivation is high.

Mindful Awareness

The topic of mindfulness was presented in Chapter Seven as a technique to help you discern between physical and emotional hunger, recognize the feelings that drive you to overeat, and become familiar with feelings of hunger and satiety. Mindfulness can also be an antidote to stress and stress-driven eating.

If you are moving quickly and distractedly on "automatic pilot" throughout the day, you are likely to feel hurried, tense, and preoccupied much of the time. You will be more likely to react to instead of respond to people and circumstances. And you will find it difficult to enjoy your life or be present for it.

If you can find ways to become more mindful, to develop moment-to-moment awareness of your surroundings and your experience of them, you can break the cycle of anxiety and irritability. The meditation techniques mentioned in Chapter Seven can help you stay present. Here are two more suggestions:

1. Take time throughout your day to slow down, breathe deeply, and pay attention. Notice your surroundings. Notice what you are feeling internally. Put this reminder on your refrigerator or computer desktop: *Stop, Breathe, Notice.*

2. Choose an activity such as brushing your teeth, washing the dishes, or walking the dog, and bring full attention to it. Just do the one thing, without distraction, and thoroughly experience it.

Nourishing Your Spirit

Quite often when I ask my clients about their daily schedules, I receive a long litany of activities that includes work, chores, errands, and childcare. Seldom is there any mention of relaxation or down time. It's not surprising that eating becomes a way of coping with an overloaded schedule filled with activities that serve everyone's needs but your own. You might be snacking in the middle of the afternoon so that you can keep moving full blast through the rest of day. Late-night snacking might be the way you reward yourself for working so hard.

The body and the mind are constantly trying to return to a state of equilibrium. If you are not taking time for yourself; if you are not creating some space and breathing room, then eating may be an unconscious way of making up for that deficit.

Here are some suggestions for replenishing your energies and creating a more balanced lifestyle:

1. Give yourself the nourishment you truly need. Read, create, listen to music, walk in nature, or do nothing at all.

Try to rest and recharge physically, mentally, and emotionally every day.

2. If you are spiritually inclined, discover or rediscover the power of prayer, meditation, or contemplation. This may or may not include participation in an organized religion.

3. Ask for help. This is hard for many of us. We are encouraged to do everything ourselves, and asking for assistance is often viewed as a sign of weakness.

   Many women have swallowed the myth that we can and should single-handedly "bring home the bacon and fry it up in a pan." A lot of women are doing it all and doing it alone. And a lot of women are very unhappy. So ask for the help you need. Learn to receive as well as you give.

Act on your own behalf. Put your needs in the foreground of your life for an established period each day. Then the need to nurture yourself with food can recede.

CALL TO ACTION:

1. Develop or continue a relaxation/meditation practice.

2. Practice deep breathing, using it throughout the day whenever you feel stressed out.

3. Use EFT whenever you feel anxious or overwhelmed.

4. Take some time every day just for you. Relax. Enjoy solitude. Do something you enjoy, that nourishes and fulfills you. Return your life to a state of balance.

5. Continue to practice mindfulness, paying close attention to your feelings and to the eating process itself. Apply EFT when appropriate.

6. Continue to listen daily to the hypnosis recording, "Freedom from Excess Weight." or to the recording of your choice. (See Appendix. You may find the recording of "Calm, Centered, and Serene" especially helpful.)

Chapter Eleven
EXERCISE—MOVE IT TO LOSE IT

Exercise is an indispensable part of any weight-loss program. By engaging in a regular fitness routine, you can burn fat, raise your metabolism, increase your body's insulin response, and burn off the stress that often leads to overeating. You can also raise your energy level, improve your mood, decrease your risk of heart disease, stroke, diabetes, osteoporosis, and certain cancers. You'll look better and you'll feel better.

In this chapter we explore:
- The benefits of exercise
- The type and amount of exercise you need to lose weight and keep it off
- Instructions for creating an effective and realistic exercise plan

Description and Benefits of Exercise

The major components of a well-rounded exercise program include aerobic exercise, resistance training, and flexibility. Below is a brief description of each, along with a list of benefits.

Aerobic Exercise
Aerobic exercise, also known as cardiovascular exercise, is any type of movement that uses the large muscle groups rhythmically and continuously, elevating the heart rate and breathing for a sustained period. Common examples include:
- Walking
- Jogging/running
- Swimming
- Rowing
- Stair climbing
- Bicycling

- Cross-country skiing
- Step, kick-boxing, and dance exercise classes
- Roller-skating

This type of activity increases the strength and efficiency of your heart and lungs, allowing the heart to pump larger volumes of oxygenated blood with less effort. Thus your resting heart rate slows down and your blood pressure decreases.

Aerobic exercise promotes circulation. It decreases overall cholesterol, raising your HDL, the so-called "good" cholesterol, and lowering your LDL, the "bad" cholesterol. It reduces circulating levels of triglycerides, lowering your risk of heart disease, stroke, arteriosclerosis, and cancer (colon and breast). If heart disease is already present, it can help to control or even reverse it.

Recent research confirms that vigorous aerobic exercise performed 30 minutes daily actually increases brain matter, both gray and white. Thus regular exercise will result in improved mental acuity and a better memory.

As for losing weight, aerobic activity burns calories, plain and simple.

Resistance Training

Resistance training (also referred to as muscle strengthening) is also tremendously important. You perform resistance-training using machines, free weights, rubber bands or rubber tubing. Engaging in this type of movement will increase muscular strength, making your day-to-day activities easier and more enjoyable. Stronger muscles improve balance and agility. Resistance training also increases bone density, reducing your risk of osteoporosis.

Resistance training is a great weight-loss aid. By increasing your muscle mass, you boost your metabolism, which is the rate at which your body burns calories. A standard three-month strength-training program will increase your resting metabolic rate (the amount of calories you burn at rest) by about seven percent.

Flexibility

Flexibility exercises increase range of motion. They improve co-ordination by allowing for freer and easier movement. Stretching improves posture and symmetry by realigning muscle. Flexibility exercises help prevent injury and muscle soreness. They decrease the risk of low-back pain, reduce muscle tension, and increase feelings of relaxation.

More Benefits

Exercise improves insulin sensitivity, increasing the body's ability to use the food you eat for fuel rather than storing it as fat. Consistent exercise also helps control blood-sugar levels, therefore decreasing the risk of Type 2 diabetes. If diabetes is already present, exercise can prevent or delay the serious vascular complications that can result from diabetes.

Regular exercise can help reduce physical discomfort, such as low-back or arthritic pain. It does this in several ways. It maintains or improves the integrity and strength of the joints. It increases range of motion. It improves posture and symmetry. It also reduces the chances of your developing or escalating the effects of kyphosis, the rounded upper back common to many older adults.

Regular exercise can improve your immune system, making you less likely to get sick. It can increase your energy, stamina, and vitality.

Exercise is a wonderful mood elevator. It decreases stress and can help combat depression. It helps you sleep more soundly. It can improve creativity and productivity. It also improves mental alertness and short-term memory.

In short, participation in a regular exercise program can greatly increase the quality of your life, allowing you to remain active and vital, alert and enthusiastic throughout your life. It can most definitely help you lose weight. Research confirms that when individuals exercise regularly, they are much more likely to maintain their weight loss.

The next few sections will answer the following questions regarding exercise and weight loss:
- How often do you need to exercise?
- How long should each exercise session be?
- How hard should you work?

These are recommendations, not rules. Make an exercise plan that is realistic for you, based on your current schedule and responsibilities. Commit to the process as best you can.

Aerobic Activity

Frequency and Duration of Aerobic Exercise Sessions

When exercising to lose weight, plan on three to five aerobic sessions per week. How long your sessions should be depends upon the intensity you work at. Aim for a caloric burn of between 250 and 300 per session. If you are walking or jogging, that's about three miles. You'll burn the same number of calories per mile regardless of speed. A brisk three-mile walk will take about 45 minutes at 15 miles an hour. A three-mile jog will take 30 minutes at 10 miles an hour. A slower 20 mph walk, more appropriate for beginners and older adults, will take approximately one hour.

If you are new to exercise, start with a 10-minute walk at a pace that is comfortable for you. Do this three times a week. Increase the amount of time you walk by two minutes each week. Be consistent and allow yourself to improve slowly and steadily.

Intensity

Although you will burn the same number of calories whether you take 10 minutes or 20 to cover a mile, you will receive the greatest health benefits if you exercise within appropriate target heart rate zones. To determine the intensity level that is optimal for you, follow these guidelines:

1. Determine your Maximum Heart Rate (MHR). This is the fastest your heart can beat. You calculate this by subtracting your age from 220.

2. Begin each work-out slowly, and progressively increase the intensity by warming up for eight to 10 minutes at 50% of your MHR.

3. After your warm-up, increase the intensity until you are working between 70% and 85% of your MHR. This is referred to as your Target Heart Rate (THR).

4. After you have worked out at this level for the intended period of time, cool down by gradually decreasing the intensity for the last five minutes of your aerobic session, returning to your warm-up intensity of about 50% MHR.

For example, if you are 45 years old, you calculate your target heart rate the following way:

Find your MHR by subtracting 220 from your age:
$$220 - 45 = 175$$

Multiply your THR by .50 to determine your warm-up and cool-down intensity levels:
$$175 \text{ x } .50 = 88$$

Multiply your THR by .70 and .85 to determine your THR:
$$175 \text{ x } .70 = 123$$
$$175 \text{ x } .85 = 149$$

In this example, your THR would be between 123 and 149.

In order to measure your pulse, you can either wear a heart rate monitor or take your pulse using the following method.

How to Take Your Pulse

1. Place the tips of your index, second, and third fingers on the palm side of your other wrist, below the base of the thumb. Or, place the tips of your index and second fingers on your lower neck, on either side of your windpipe.

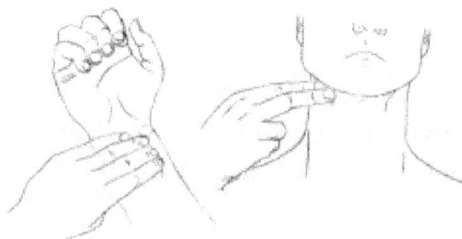

2. Press lightly with your fingers until you feel the blood pulsing beneath them. You might need to move your fingers around, slightly up or down until you feel the pulsing.

3. Use a watch with a second hand, or look at a clock with a second hand.

4. For 10 seconds, count how many beats you feel. Multiply that number by six to obtain your heart rate (pulse), per minute.

Check your pulse   x 6 =

_____   _____
(no. of beats in 10   (your pulse)
   seconds)

A simplified version of this process appears in the following chart.

Age	50% THR	10-sec	70%–85% THR	10-sec
20	100	23	140 -170	23
25	98	16	137 - 166	23 - 28
30	95	16	133 - 162	22 - 27
35	93	15	130 - 157	22 - 26
40	90	15	126 - 153	21 - 26
45	88	15	123 - 149	20 - 25
50	85	14	119 - 145	20 - 24
55	83	14	116 - 140	19 - 23
60	80	13	112 - 136	19 - 23
65	78	13	109 - 132	18 - 22
70	75	13	105 - 128	18 - 21
75	73	12	102 - 123	17 - 21
80	70	12	98 - 119	16 - 20
85	68	11	95 - 115	16 - 19
90	65	11	91 - 111	15 - 18

Perceived Rate of Exertion (PRE)

Another useful tool for measuring appropriate intensity is the Perceived Rate of Exertion Scale. It is especially useful for older adults, since many of the commonly prescribed medications for this age group, such as beta-blockers and digitalis drugs, lower the heart rate.

By tuning into how hard or easy you feel you're working, you can regulate and maintain the proper level of intensity.

Level #1: This is the feeling you have when you are at rest. There is no feeling of fatigue, and your breathing is even and steady.

Level #2: This is the feeling you might have while getting dressed. There is little or no feeling of fatigue, and your breathing is even and steady.

Level #3: This is the feeling you might have while slowly walking across the room to turn on the T.V. There is little feeling of fatigue. You might be slightly aware of your breathing, but it is slow and natural.

Level #4: This is the feeling you might have while slowly walking outside. There is a very slight feeling of effort. Your breathing is slightly elevated, but comfortable. You might experience this level during the initial stages of your warm-up.

Level #5: This is the feeling you might have while walking briskly to the store. There is a slight feeling of fatigue. You are aware of your breathing and it is deeper than in level 4. *You should experience this level during your warm-up.*

Level #6: This is the feeling you might have when you are walking briskly somewhere for more than a few minutes and are very late for an appointment. There is a general feeling of fatigue, but you know that you can maintain this level. Your breathing is somewhat deep and you are aware of it beginning to feel labored. *You should experience this level during the transition from your warm-up to your baseline work-out level.*

Level #7: This is the feeling you might have as you begin to increase your exercise intensity. You feel challenged, but can maintain this level for the rest of your exercise session. Your breathing is deep. You can carry on a conversation, but would probably prefer not to. *This is the baseline working level that you want to achieve during an exercise session.*

Level #8: This is the feeling you might have when you are exercising very vigorously and "in the zone." You can probably continue at this intensity, but it is quite challenging. Your breathing is very deep; you can still carry on a conversation, but you probably won't feel like it. At this level you are working hard and feeling challenged. *This is the feeling you should experience only after you have become comfortable reaching a level 7 and are ready for a more intense work-out.*

Level #9: This is the feeling that you would experience if you were exercising very, very vigorously, just short of an all-out sprint. Your breathing is heavy and labored. It would be very difficult or impossible to carry on a conversation. You should not be experiencing a level 9, even for short time periods, unless you are engaged in interval training (see below).

Level #10: This is the feeling you would experience with all-out exertion. This level cannot be maintained for very long, possibly not more than 30 seconds. This is not a training level and there is no benefit in reaching it unless you are a competitive athlete (or are performing a stress test in a doctor's office).

To use this scale, observe how your body feels, how hard you are breathing, and how hard your muscles are working as you move through increasing levels of exertion. With practice, you will be able to gauge intensity levels with a fair amount of accuracy. If you multiply a level number by 10, it will approximate the corresponding percentage of your maximum heart rate. For example, if you are exercising at a perceived intensity level of 5 and you multiply that by 10, you are probably working at 50% of your maximum heart rate.

Walking Programs
Walking is the most popular type of aerobic exercise. And for good reason. It is simple, uncomplicated, inexpensive, and often quite enjoyable, especially when the weather is pleasant and you

can walk in natural surroundings. In the appendix are several walking and jogging programs of varying levels and intensities.

If you routinely walk on flat surfaces, you will eventually need to increase your intensity level. You can do this in one these ways:

- Climb hills if you're walking outdoors.
- Add weight. (I recommend a weighted vest; hand-held dumbbells can put you at risk for shoulder injury.)
- Raise the level of incline if you're on a treadmill.
- Jog or perform walk/jog intervals.

You will find progressive walking and jogging programs on the **"Resources"** page of my website: *www.tlcweightloss.net/resources.php*

Interval Training

One of the best ways to rev up the fat-burning capacity of an aerobic routine is to engage in interval training. Not only will you burn more calories during your workout, you will continue to do so for several hours afterward.

Intervals can be performed whether you swim, walk, run, or do any other aerobic exercise. There are different interval programs that serve various goals. For weight loss, follow these guidelines:

1. Warm up 8–10 minutes at 50% to 60% of your MHR before starting intervals.

2. Perform the high-intensity intervals at 85% to 95% MHR.

3. Perform the moderate-intensity intervals at 70% to 80% MHR.

4. The ratio of high-to-moderate-intensity intervals will be 3:1 initially. For example, you will perform 90 seconds of moderate-intensity exercise for every 30 seconds at a high intensity. Gradually work up to a 2:1 ratio.

5. Cool down for 5 minutes.

Here is a sample interval training program:

35-Minute Interval Training Program

10-minute warm-up at 50% to 60% MHR

Perform 10 intervals of the following:
30-second high-intensity interval at 85% to 90 % MHR
followed by
90-second moderate-intensity interval at 70% to 80% MHR

5-minute cool-down

Resistance Training

As stated previously, increasing muscle mass will rev up your metabolism, boosting your body's capacity to burn calories, even at rest. And if you don't intentionally build muscle while losing weight, you run the risk of losing lean muscle mass as well as fat, thereby slowing down your metabolism.

For optimal weight loss, perform muscle-strengthening exercises at least two times per week on alternate days. Use free weights, machines, rubber tubing, body weight, or any combination of these. You can hit all the major muscle groups, performing two sets of each exercise, in about 30 minutes.

Weight-Training Guidelines

To execute a resistance-training routine that is safe and effective, follow these guidelines.

Warm up. Warming up promotes safety, prevents injury, and increases performance. Before beginning your weightlifting session, do some form of cardiovascular exercise at a light, comfortable intensity for about five to 10 minutes. Walking or riding a bicycle works well.

Select at least one exercise for each major muscle group in order to promote well-balanced muscle development. That means choosing at least one exercise for each of the following groups:

- Chest
- Upper back
- Biceps
- Triceps
- Shoulders
- Gluteus Maximus
- Quadriceps
- Hamstrings
- Core: abdomen and lower back

Perform your exercises in the optimal sequence. When performing a variety of weightlifting exercises, it is advisable to proceed from the larger muscle groups to the smaller ones. This allows optimal performance of the most demanding exercises when fatigue levels are the lowest and you feel fresh.

If you are working your upper body, begin by working your chest and back muscles, followed by shoulders, biceps, and triceps. If working the lower body, work the gluteus maximus, followed by the quadriceps and hamstrings.

Perform two to three sets of each exercise. A set is the number of successive repetitions performed without resting.

Perform eight to 15 repetitions in each set. There are many different ways to mix repetitions and sets, and the optimal mix depends upon your goals. The following method will provide a safe and effective workout for overall fitness and weight loss.

Use a relatively light weight for the first set and perform 12 to 15 repetitions. Choose a weight for your next set that will fatigue your muscles in eight to 12 repetitions. Do this by increasing the resistance by five to 10 percent. This is called muscle overload, and it will make all the difference between maintaining your current level of strength and increasing it. If you perform a third set, increase the resistance again and perform six to 10 repetitions Rest for 30 to 60 seconds in between each set.

To Summarize:

- Work all the major muscle groups, starting with the larger ones.
- Perform two to three sets of each exercise.
    1. First set—Perform 12–15 repetitions.
    2. Second set—Increase resistance by approximately 5% to 10%. Perform 10 to 12 repetitions.
    3. Third set—Increase the resistance again, as above, and perform six to 10 repetitions.
- Rest for 30 to 60 seconds between each set.

The Overload Principle refers to the fact that the body will adapt to stresses placed upon it. When you stress the body by lifting a weight heavier than the body is unaccustomed to lifting, the body reacts by becoming stronger in order to handle that stress the next time it occurs.

Progressive resistance is imperative for overloading the muscle. As your muscles adapt to a given exercise resistance (weight), that resistance must be gradually increased to stimulate further gains. This requires the gradual and continual addition of weight to the exercise over time. As the weights become too easy to lift, change to heavier ones so that your body is continually forced to work harder and thus increase muscle strength, size, and tone.

Move slowly. Fast lifting creates momentum. Move slowly and your muscles will be more effectively challenged. Speed also increases your risk of injury.

Use proper form and technique. The most common and critical training mistakes may be those of exercise technique. The tendency to use too much weight before your body is ready for it typically results in poor form, which decreases your ability to get results, and increases the risk of injury. When strengthening the muscles, you must isolate the movement to that particular muscle group. This is not how we move during our daily activities, and it may feel awkward at first. Give yourself time to learn proper technique before you increase the amount of resistance you are lifting.

Exercise through a full range of motion. Perform each exercise through the full range of motion that muscle group is capable of.

Train every other day. Resistance training produces tissue microtrauma—tiny tears in the muscles that temporarily decrease strength and cause varying degrees of muscle soreness. Muscles generally require about 48 hours for the resting and rebuilding process before you work them again. It is during this rest and repair period that the muscles actually become bigger and stronger. Two to three muscle training sessions a week are enough to build strength if your goal is overall fitness.

Change your routine regularly. To avoid plateaus and to head off boredom, it is best to change your muscle strengthening routine every six to eight weeks.

Stretch after each resistance-training session. When you strengthen your muscles, you shorten them. Take the time to redress this shortening by stretching and lengthening all major muscles after your resistance training. Hold each stretch for 20 to 30 seconds.

On my website you will find a comprehensive resistance-training program. Go to the "**Resources**" page of my website: *www.tlcweightloss.net/resources.php*

Body Mass Index vs. Body Fat Percentage

As stated previously, if you don't perform resistance-training exercises, you may lose lean muscle mass as well as fat, thereby slowing down your metabolism. Therefore your goal should be to *lose fat* and *retain* or *gain muscle.*

Increasing muscle mass increases the energy-burning capacity of your body. You will lose weight faster, and the probability of remaining at your ideal weight will increase.

The Body Mass Index, or BMI, is a measurement of body weight relative to height, and is often referred to when assessing ideal weight. However, BMI does not distinguish between fat and lean body mass. People with large amounts of lean tissue may have a high BMI although their body fat percentage is in a healthy range. Conversely, a low BMI does not necessarily mean that body fat is within a healthy range.

Body fat, not weight, is a better measure of your health and fitness. Because the scale does not distinguish between lean weight and fat weight, a person could be "over-weight" but not be "over-fat." The reverse is also true.

Body fat can be measured in several ways. The most common methods are through the use of skinfold calipers or a Bioelectrical Impedance (BEI) Analyzer. Each method has a margin of error of approximately 3–5%.

A personal trainer at your local gym can assess your body fat percentage with one of these two methods. You can also purchase a scale that measures BEI. According to About.com, the most accurate and reliable scales as of this date are listed below. You can access their website here: http://walking.about.com/od/calorie1/tp/bodyfatmonitor.htm:

1. Tanita BF-682 Scale and Body Fat Monitor
2. Omron Body Fat Analyzer
3. FatTrack Digital Skinfold Caliper

The body fat percentage guidelines listed below can give you a general framework to work within.

Women

Age	Underfat	Healthy Range	Overweight	Obese
20–40 yrs	Under 21%	21–33%	33–39%	Over 39%
41–60 yrs	Under 23%	23–35%	35–40%	Over 40%
61–79 yrs	Under 24%	24–36%	36–42%	Over 42%

Men

Age	Underfat	Healthy Range	Overweight	Obese
20–40 yrs	Under 8%	8–19%	19–25%	Over 25%
41–60 yrs	Under 11%	11–22%	22–27%	Over 27%
61–79 yrs	Under 13%	13–25%	25–30%	Over 30%

Flexibility

Stretching counterbalances the more vigorous forms of exercise by stretching the muscles that have been contracted and thus shortened during exercise. Although stretching will not directly contribute to weight loss, it is important to the safety and overall effectiveness of your exercise program. It will improve the range of motion in your joints, improve circulation, decrease muscle soreness, and reduce the risk of injury.

Stretching is most effective at the end of your aerobic and resistance-training routine when the muscles are warm and blood is circulating freely through them. Take about five minutes after each workout to stretch each major muscle group, holding each stretch for 20 to 30 seconds.

You will find a comprehensive flexibility program on the "**Resources**" page of my website:
www.tlcweightloss.net/resources.php

Medical Considerations

It is always a good idea to check with your doctor before you begin a regular exercise program. It is especially important to do so if you answer *yes* to any of these questions.

1. Are you a man over 40 or a woman over 50?

2. Do you have two or more of these risk factors?
   - Family history of heart attack or sudden death
   - Current cigarette smoking
   - High blood pressure
   - High cholesterol
   - Diabetes
   - Physical inactivity

3. Have you been told you have a heart condition and should only participate in physical activity recommended by a doctor?

4. Do you feel pain (or discomfort) in your chest when you do physical activity? When you are not participating in

physical activity? While at rest, do you frequently experience fast, irregular heartbeats or very slow beats?

5. Do you ever become dizzy and lose your balance, or lose consciousness? Have you fallen more than twice in the past year (regardless of the reason)?

6. Do you have a bone or joint problem that could worsen as a result of physical activity? Do you have pain in your legs or buttocks when you walk?

7. Do you take blood pressure or heart medication?

8. Do you have any cuts or wounds on your feet that don't seem to heal?

9. Have you experienced unexplained weight loss in the past six months?

If you answered *no* to all of these questions, you can be reasonably sure that you can safely take part in at least a moderate physical activity program. But if you answered *yes* to any of them, check with your physician before getting started.

Exercise Tips

Here are a few things to keep in mind as you embark upon an exercise program:

- **Get proper instruction.** Find a qualified fitness professional who can teach you proper technique (see Appendix), or work out with an experienced training partner.
- **Start slowly.** One of the most common mistakes new exercisers make is taking on too much too fast. Begin with short bouts of moderate exercise and gradually increase the time and intensity of your workouts. Allow your body

time to adjust to the challenge. You will reduce your risk of injury, feel more successful, and increase the likelihood of sticking with it.

- **Set realistic goals.** Having clear objectives and challenging but achievable goals will motivate you to get to the gym or take that afternoon walk on days when you just want to lie down on the couch.

- **Choose a workout you enjoy.** 30 minutes on the treadmill is torture if you'd rather be walking outdoors or taking a group exercise class. It's crucial to choose some activity you enjoy doing. Otherwise you'll dread exercise, and it will be difficult to maintain your enthusiasm.

- **Be consistent.** Work out at the same time each day if possible, choosing a time that suits you best. That may be first thing in the morning, mid afternoon, right after work, or after dinner. The idea is to develop an exercise "habit" so that you integrate fitness smoothly into your life. When you do this, you will find that you actually miss exercising if you skip a session.

- **Fit in fitness whenever possible.** Three 10–minute exercise sessions can be almost as beneficial as one 30-minute workout. If you can't do your workout in one session, break it up into shorter sessions throughout the day. You might get off the bus one stop early, walk to the office or supermarket, or walk through the park at lunchtime.

- **Find an exercise partner.** Make two appointments per week to meet up with someone and exercise. If you have a friend relying on you to go to the gym or take a morning walk with her/him, you'll be less likely to cancel. Write down any workout dates in your diary and commit to them as if they were business meetings.

- **Vary your fitness activity.** Changing your routine frequently will stave off boredom. It will also prevent fitness plateaus. Cross-train by incorporating a variety of strength training, flexibility, and cardiovascular exercises into your routine. Incorporate a yoga or Pilates class. Try a new group exercise class. Take up skating or tennis.

- **Skip a day.** Allowing your muscles to rest and rejuvenate is a crucial part of being healthy and achieving maximum results. Giving yourself a break now and then prevents burn-out and makes you more likely to stick to a long-term exercise plan. Listen to your body, and if you're having an off day, take it easy and rest.
- **Always have a Plan B available.** Life happens. Be prepared with an alternative to your original plan. Keep socks and a pair of walking shoes in your car. If you don't have 45 minutes available for exercise that day, try to accrue at least 30 minutes throughout the day, and find more time to exercise the following day.

Creating an Exercise Plan

There are a number of things to consider when designing your exercise program. Begin by asking yourself some questions:
- What kind of activities do I enjoy?
- Do I want to exercise inside or out?
- Do I prefer the gym or would I rather work out at home?
- Do I enjoy exercising with a partner or in a group, or do I prefer to work out alone?
- When is the best time for me to exercise?

For the aerobic portion of your exercise program, list physical activities that you enjoy. Some possibilities include walking, swimming, bicycling, dancing, or joining a group exercise class.

_____

_____

_____

_____

_____

Next, plan your resistance-training routine. Consider the following options:

- Work out at home. You can use home gym equipment, free weights, videos, personal training, etc.
- Go to a gym. You can use machines or free weights. You can also join a group exercise class.

Write down your preferences.

_____

_____

_____

_____

The next question is, when are you going to work out? Here are some possibilities:

- If you work outside the home, you can exercise before work, afterwards, or during lunch.
- If you are caring for young children, you will need to work around their needs and schedules. You might exercise in the morning before they get up, during their afternoon naps, or after dinner.

The length of your workout is also a factor. Think about the following options:

- Combine your aerobic and resistance-training routines in the same session. Ideally, these sessions will be 45 minutes to an hour, three or four times a week. You can divide your strength-training sessions, performing upper body exercises during one workout and lower body and core exercises during another.
- Alternate aerobic and resistance-training sessions. These will take 30 to 35 minutes, five to six times per week.
- Break up your workouts into 10 or 20-minute sessions throughout the day.

Record your preferences.

_____

_____

_____

_____

Now write two exercise plans for the week. One will include your preferred choice of time, place, and type of exercise. The second will be for when there are obstacles to your original plan.

	Plan A	Plan B
Monday	Walk 35 min. on treadmill.	Walk to the office from the bus stop: 15 min. Walk at lunch time: 20 min.
Tuesday	Go to gym after work; weight train for 30 min., 20 min. on elliptical trainer.	Use weight training/step video at home.
Wednesday	Swim for 35 min. after dinner.	Take dog for extra long walk: 35 min.
Thursday	Go to gym for one hour and work with personal trainer.	Do body weight exercises at home, such as push-ups, sit-ups, chair dips, squats. Add jumping jacks and jumping rope.
Friday	Attend aerobic class.	Take your bicycle out for a spin around the neighborhood.
Saturday	Attend a yoga class	Use a video to do yoga.
Sunday	Hike or bike with family members.	Go to the local YMCA and join a family swim.

Now it is your turn.

	Plan A	Plan B
Monday		
Tuesday		
Wednesday		
Thursday		
Friday		
Saturday		
Sunday		

To increase your level of commitment and accountability, fill out the following contract for the week ahead; write down what you plan to do on each day, sign it, then have a witness sign it (preferably someone who cares about and supports your healthy weight-loss efforts). Then, each time you complete an exercise session, record your accomplishments. Remember, if something comes between you and your original plan, refer to Plan B. You will find a copy of this contract on the "**Resources**" page of my website: *www.tlcweightloss.net/resources.php*

WEEKLY PERSONAL FITNESS CONTRACT

I, _____, accept my responsibility to comply with the following exercise program in order to achieve my fitness goals of weight loss, increased strength, endurance, vitality, and overall health.

	Plan	Actual
Monday		
Tuesday		
Wednesday		
Thursday		
Friday		
Saturday		
Sunday		

Signed _____

Witnessed by _____

Workout Logs

It is important to keep a written record of your workouts. A workout log will help you keep track of what you do in each exercise session and chart your progress.

Keep two exercise logs. One will include general information about your exercise session, such as the following:
- Date
- Type of activity
- Time spent
- Intensity level

A resistance-training log should record the following:
- Type of exercise
- Number of sets
- Amount of resistance

You will find two exercise logs on the "**Resources**" page of my website: _www.tlcweightloss.net/resources.php_ It can also be helpful to record how you feel about your exercise session, especially if you are feeling stuck or unmotivated. Here are some suggestions:
- Write about how the exercise session felt that day.
- Write about your personal thoughts and feelings regarding your progress.
- Create affirmations or positive, motivating statements.
- Write about acceptance, challenge, fear, and success.

Personal Training

If you need assistance learning exercise technique, creating an exercise plan, or any issues regarding fitness, hire a personal trainer. He or she will work with you to create a program that takes into account your goals, interests, schedule, preferences, and current fitness level. A trainer will also teach you how to exercise in the safest and most effective manner, providing education, motivation and accountability. You can find lists of certified personal trainers at the American College of Sports Medicine (ACSM) and the American Council on Exercise (ACE) websites. See the "Recommended Resources" section of the Appendix.

EFT for Resistance to Exercise

You may find yourself resisting the idea of beginning a fitness program. Or maybe you exercise but are not consistent. Use EFT to tap away all of your reasons and excuses for not exercising.

"Even though I don't have time to exercise..."

"Even though I don't like to exercise..."

"Even though I'm too tired to exercise..."

Tune into the level of your resistance, as well as any self-judgment that might arise around this issue. Tap until your intensity level is a 2 or lower on the SUDs scale. Then create your exercise plan, and move forward.

CALL TO ACTION

1. Make a list of exercises you enjoy doing, decide on the optimal time and place to exercise, create an exercise plan and execute it. Don't forget to have a Plan B available.

2. Use EFT to eliminate any resistance you may have to exercising, as well as for food cravings, the emotional distress that prompt overeating, and any resistance to the weight-loss process that crops up.

3. Continue to practice mindfulness, paying close attention to your feelings and to the eating process itself. Apply EFT when appropriate.

4. Take time each day to relax. Find adequate down time. Do things that you enjoy. Find balance in your life, and guard it carefully.

5. Continue to listen daily to the hypnosis recording, "Freedom from Excess Weight." or to the recording of your choosing. (See Appendix. You may find the hypnosis recording of "Exercise Motivation" especially helpful.)

Chapter Twelve
CONTINUED SUCCESS

This chapter contains some final thoughts on the major topics covered in this book. It offers suggestions for handling the inevitable slips and plateaus that occur during the weight-loss process. It includes typical sabotaging thoughts and feelings that might arise and how you can handle them with EFT. And it presents challenging scenarios that might crop up as you continue to move through your weight-loss journey, coupled with ways to manage them successfully.

<u>Final Thoughts</u>

Nutrition
Eat some combination of high-quality protein, nourishing fats, fruits and vegetables, and a limited amount of high-fiber starchy carbohydrates like oatmeal and sweet potatoes. Experiment with combinations, and discover what works best for you.

Exercise
Create a schedule that is realistic and doable. Exercise can improve your health, your mood and energy level, diminish your stress, and lower your weight. If these benefits could be put in a pill, we would all most certainly take it daily. But they can't. So get moving. The payback for this kind of effort is immeasurable.

Mindfulness
Consume your meals slowly, with awareness, and you will enjoy them much more. And here's the paradox: enjoy your food this way and you are less likely to overeat. You can experience the delight of consuming really tasty, healthy food, and allow eating to take its place as one of life's great pleasures.

Pay attention to your life, not just your food intake. Be present for all your experiences. Doing so can bring tremendous joy and peace.

Stress
Slow down as best you can, and create some space for yourself. Self-care is not just about the discipline of eating well and exercising. It is about allowing adequate time for those activities that nurture, replenish, and sustain you.

Resistance
Expect it. It is an inherent part of the weight-loss process. Work with the part of you that does not want to change. Respect that part. Be tolerant and compassionate toward yourself. Self-loathing is not helpful. It only locks the resistance in place.

Healing the Past
Even if your past has not directly contributed to your present food struggles, it is still a good idea to do some emotional clearing with EFT. Consider using Gary Craig's Peace Procedure, mentioned in Chapter Nine. There is great serenity and spiritual balance inherent in this kind of work.

Get help! If your past was indeed difficult; if you grew up in a dysfunctional environment; if you suffered physical and/or emotional abuse, do not try to work through these issues on your own. Find a compassionate and knowledgeable therapist, ideally one who uses EFT. Know that healing is possible, and allow the pain to be your gateway to healing.

EFT and Hypnosis
Continue to practice self-hypnosis and EFT every day. Not just for weight loss, but for any goal you have set before you—for any situation that causes stress or inner turmoil—for anything that stands between you and inner peace, contentment and joy.

Falling Off the Diet Wagon

There will be times during this weight-loss journey when you may find yourself regaining some of the weight you have lost. When stressful situations crop up—and they will—you may fall back on old coping mechanisms such as overeating. Or the holidays will come around, and you could find yourself falling into old patterns of eating way too much of the wrong foods. Or you might go on vacation and watch your carefully crafted eating plan fly right out the window.

Don't panic. The problem is not the slip into old eating patterns, but how you interpret it.

You may berate yourself, telling yourself you have no willpower, that you are weak and stupid, and you will never succeed. You may find yourself thinking, "Oh well, I blew it; I might as well eat whatever I want." This kind of thinking can propel you onto the slippery slope of steady weight gain.

Reality check—you gained a pound or two. Guilt and self-loathing will do much more harm to your weight-loss efforts than the actual weight gain will.

The Solution

Endeavor to see this event as an inevitable stumbling block that everyone hits, not evidence of failure. Here are a few tips:

1. Recognize that an occasional slip is a very normal part of the weight-loss process. As much as you'd like to, you can't live in a bubble while you're trying to lose weight. Life happens.

2. Use EFT for forgiveness and self-acceptance. You may find one or more of the following statements helpful:

"Even though I feel awful for eating_____, I deeply and completely love, accept, and forgive myself."

"Even though I don't deserve to let myself off the hook, I recognize that beating myself up is not helpful; it actually makes losing weight harder, so I'm willing to accept myself and all of my mistakes."

"Even though I feel really stupid for eating _____; I know better; what's wrong with me? I deeply and completely accept myself anyway."

"Even though it feels so hard to go back to my food plan, I recognize and honor how difficult this is, and I accept myself and my struggles."

3. Return to your weight-loss plan. If that is too difficult…

4. Get help. At the risk of sounding like a broken record, sometimes you simply cannot take this on by yourself. Find a support group. Or seek out a professional Weight-Loss Coach. I am available for this type of assistance, in person or by phone, and you can email me at *terry@tlcweightloss.net*. Or find a qualified EFT practitioner in your area.

Remember, departing from your food plan is not the problem. Perceiving it as personal failure is. Forgive yourself. Let it go. And then move forward.

Plateaus

Like the occasional slips when you regain weight, plateaus are a frustrating but probably unavoidable part of the weight-loss process. Do not panic. Below are some possible causes, followed by methods you can use to refocus.

There are several reasons why you might find your weight loss stalled. Here are a few:

Cause: You are losing fat and gaining muscle. This, of course, is ideal. As stated in Chapter Eleven, increase your muscle mass and you increase your metabolism.
Solution: If your scale isn't moving but your clothes fit better, then this is probably the case. To make sure, check your body percentage and take your measurements, as suggested in Chapter One.

Cause: You are retaining water. If you don't drink enough water, your body will hold onto the water it does have, and fluid retention can result.
Solution: Drink at least six to eight glasses of water a day. Some medications can also cause water retention, so if you are on any prescription medications, ask your doctor about this possibility.

Cause: Your body is going through a period of adjustment. When you lose weight, your body operates something like the feedback loop of a thermostat. It needs periods of adjustment to catch up with the different amount and type of fuel it is getting, just as a thermostat needs to "catch up" with changes in the temperature inside your home.
Solution: Be patient. If you're resetting your "set point," it happens in stages. Being stuck at a certain weight for a few weeks may just be your body's way of reprogramming itself.

Cause: You are eating too many carbohydrates. The consequences of consuming too many starchy carbohydrates have been discussed at length in this manual. And you may be more sensitive than most.
Solution: Pull all starchy carbohydrates—all grains, sugar and high-glycemic vegetables (potatoes, corn, peas), out of your diet for a week or two. Then slowly add them back and note

the results, so you can figure out the amount of carbohydrate consumption that is best for you.

Cause: You aren't eating enough protein. If you don't eat enough protein, your body will break down its own muscle mass for fuel. If this happens, you will lose muscle, thus lowering your metabolic rate.

Solution: Make sure that at least 25% of your caloric intake comes from high-quality sources of protein such as fish, chicken, beef, beans, and whey protein powder.

Cause: You are overeating. Even if you make healthy food choices most of the time, you will still gain weight if you are eating too much food overall.

Solution: Refer to Chapter Five, study the food exchange tables, and figure out how much you should be eating. You may need to weigh and measure your food for awhile, just to get a realistic view of how much you are really consuming. Refer to Chapter Seven on Mindful Eating. Be sure you are eating only when you are physically hungry, and stop when you are comfortably full.

Cause: You are undereating. When you don't eat enough—under 1,000 calories daily—your metabolism slows down in order to use incoming fuel more efficiently.

Solution: Eat when you are hungry, stop when you are full, and eat enough to sustain your daily activity levels. This will require at least 1,200 calories a day.

Cause: You are not exercising. Although you can lose weight without exercising, you will lose it faster if you do. In addition, without regular resistance training, you will lose both muscle and fat. Then, if you regain the weight, you will gain only fat.

Solution: You know what to do!

Cause: You have stopped using hypnosis and/or EFT. You let go of your daily self-hypnosis sessions because you didn't think you needed them anymore. Or you forgot to tap.

Solution: If you are struggling, find your favorite hypnosis CD and listen to it every day. Or find another hypnosis CD, created either by me or by another hypnotherapist. Use it regularly to get back on track. A live hypnosis session can also be very effective. Return to a daily EFT practice. Go back to the basics, tapping to decrease your strongest food cravings. Working in person with a qualified EFT practitioner can also be extremely helpful. Revisit Chapter Five for other possibilities. These include:

- Food sensitivities
- Medications
- Birth control pills
- Low-functioning thyroid gland

EFT: Imagining the Future

Below are possible objections or negative beliefs you may have when you imagine your future as a thinner person who consistently makes healthy food choices. Possible choice statements have been incorporated. Use them if they resonate with you, or create your own.

Sabotaging Beliefs
See if any of these statements reflect your feelings or beliefs. If so, tap daily until you have vanquished them. Do not allow self-sabotage to ruin the great strides you have made so far.

Picture yourself at your goal weight. How do you feel?

"Even though I can't believe I will really be thin, I choose to believe that I can actually do this."

"Even though I don't think I can keep the weight off because I never have before, I choose to know with certainty that this time it is possible."

"Even though I find it hard to imagine myself as a thin person, I choose to let it be easy."

"Even though being thin makes me nervous, I choose to feel safe and secure."

Preparing for Future Events

1. Imagine yourself in a stressful or emotionally difficult situation and *not* turning to food. How do you feel?

"Even though I'm worried that I can't handle stress without food, I choose to feel calm and confident."

"Even though I may still want to eat when I feel anxious, angry, pressured, tired, or bored, I choose to remember that I can tap away any uncomfortable feelings."

2. Imagine yourself at a holiday or family gathering.

"Even though I always overeat at Thanksgiving (Passover, Christmas, etc.), I choose to know that this time will be different."

"Even though I feel guilty if I don't eat my mother's cooking..."

"Even though I can't pass up all those goodies..."

3. What other future situations might trigger the urge to overeat?

"Even though I tend to overeat whenever I go out to dinner, I choose to stop eating when I am comfortably full."

"Even though I always eat too much when I'm at my mother's house, I choose to eat slowly and mindfully so I know when I've had enough."

"Even though I want to overeat as I get closer to my goal weight, I choose to remain focused on what I truly want."

"Even though I'm afraid I'll gain the weight back because I always have before, I choose to feel excited because I know this time I can succeed!"

Going Forth

As you work on neutralizing emotional distress and any childhood memories that have fueled overeating, you will become a calmer, happier person. Joy will replace discomfort. Serenity may replace anxiety. These may be new feelings for you. Get used to them. You have begun to heal, and there's no going back.

And here's one more bit of advice:

Do one exquisitely kind thing for yourself every day!

Take a warm bath, read a good book, or sit and do nothing at all. Buy yourself flowers, listen to beautiful music, or spend time on your favorite hobby. Enjoy a walk in the woods, a day in the garden, or a weekend at the beach.

Take care of yourself. Be kind to yourself. Nourish yourself with what you truly need, including healthy, nutritious food. Then eating will take its rightful place as just one of life's many pleasures.

Endnotes

[1] *American Journal of Clinical Nutrition,* January 13, 2010.

[2] National Center for Health Statistics, *Survey of Mortality Rates,* (Hyattsville, MD: 2008).

[3] *The New York Times,* February 6, 2004.

[4] "NUTRITION: The Soft Science of Dietary Fat," *Science,* 291 (March 30, 2001).

[5] *The New York Times,* July 7, 2002.

[6] *Journal of Medicine,* July 17, 2008.

[7] Green, P. Pilot 12-week feeding weight loss comparison: low fat vs. low carbohydrate diets. Abstact 95. Presented at the North American Association for the Study of Obesity's 2003 Annual Meeting.

[8] *www.health.gov/dietaryguidelines/dga2005/document/pdf/dga2005.pdf*

APPENDICES

Appendix A: TLC WEIGHT LOSS SERVICES

Terry L Currier offers **Weight-Loss Coaching** in person and by phone. These sessions provide:

- A nutritional program to help you lose weight while elevating mood, boosting energy, and improving overall health
- An exercise program that is safe, effective and realistic
- Instruction in the use of EFT to eliminate food cravings and neutralize the emotions that prompt overeating
- Live hypnosis sessions, recorded on CDs for home use, to make lifestyle changes required to lose weight much easier, while keeping you focused and motivated
- The utilization of EFT to explore and heal emotional issues that promote overeating, change negative beliefs that sabotage weight loss, and break through resistance to being thinner and/or eating differently
- Instruction in the use of mindfulness to increase awareness of hunger and satiety signals and tune into feelings that prompt overeating
- Instruction and practice of stress management techniques to reduce the anxiety and agitation that may drive overeating
- Hypnosis sessions to make the required lifestyle changes easier and to heal the emotional issues that may prompt overeating
- Support, guidance, motivation, and accountability

Visit my website for more information and current pricing: *www.tlcweightloss.net/services_and_programs.php*

Free Strategy Sessions

If you'd like to learn more about TLC Weight Loss Coaching, I offer a free 30-minute Strategy Session. In this conversation, which we'll have by phone, we will explore your history, your current concerns, and your goals regarding weight loss. I will give you suggestions and strategies for achieving those goals. If you wish to pursue further sessions, we'll discuss how TLC Weight Loss Coaching can help. I will provide you with lots of clear information and guidance and will never pressure you to purchase my services. Call **(781) 690-6112** or email: _terry@tlcweightloss.net_.

TLC Weight Loss Groups

I facilitate live weight-loss groups in the Boston, MA area. These groups have between six and 10 participants, and draw upon the information and practices espoused in _Waist Management_. The meetings incorporate the following:

- Discussions concerning the progress, issues, and concerns of each participant
- Educational lectures pertaining to nutrition, exercise, mindfulness, stress, and emotional eating
- Instructions for applying EFT to the issues that arise during the weight-loss process
- A group hypnosis session related to the topic or theme of the meeting

See my website for current schedule:
_www.tlcweightloss.net/services_and_programs.php_

Coming in June of 2012:

WAIST MANAGEMENT COMPANION

This downloadable ebook expands upon the information provided in *Waist Management*. It includes the following:

- An expanded food exchange list
- An expanded glycemic load list
- Instructions for reading food labels
- More meal and snack ideas
- Recipes
- Weight Loss for Warriors—my own low-carb diet plan
- In-depth instruction for crafting EFT statements
- More detailed information regarding Gary Craig's Personal Peace Procedure
- Descriptions of various meditation techniques and mindfulness practices
- Detailed instruction on creating your own self-hypnosis scripts
- More resistance training routines
- Expanded logs and journal for food, exercise, and EFT statements
- Detailed Q and A

And much, much more!

Appendix B: WAIST MANAGEMENT HYPNOSIS RECORDINGS

Freedom from Excess Weight

Click on the link below to receive this free hypnosis recording:
www.tlcweightloss.net/bonus.php

On a PC right-click the link **"Freedom from Excess Weight"** and hit Save Target As. On a Mac, click the link. After the file opens, save it to your computer. This will allow you to burn it to a blank CD or download it onto an ipod or mp3 player.

This recording contains motivational messages and suggestions that include:
- Making appropriate lifestyle changes such as eating well and exercising
- Imagining how great you will look and feel at your ideal weight
- Practicing self-care

As suggested throughout the book, listen to this recording daily for optimal effectiveness.

To assist in your weight-loss efforts, I have created additional hypnosis recordings, which are listed below. They can be purchased as CDs or downloadable mp3 files from the TLC Weight Loss website: www.tlcweightloss.net/products.php

"Eat, Drink and Be Healthy"
Listening to this recording will reinforce your desire to eat well, choosing fresh fruits and vegetables, whole grains, lean protein, and healthy fat. It will also encourage you to drink generous amounts of water.

"Mindful Eating"

This hypnosis session will help you pay attention to hunger and satiety signals so that you will eat only when you are physically hungry and stop when you feel full. It emphasizes slow and mindful food consumption so that you actually enjoy your meals and can easily stop eating when you have had enough.

"Healing the Hungry Heart"

With this recording you will use your imagination to create a hunger and satiety scale, eating only when you are hungry and stopping when you have had enough. You will be encouraged to take care of your true needs so that you don't stuff your feelings and needs down with food. And it will inspire you to use EFT to neutralize the uncomfortable emotions that might drive you to overeat.

"Exercise Motivation"

As the name implies, this hypnosis recording will inspire you to move. It will create in you an eagerness to exercise so that you actually look forward to your workouts.

"Calm, Centered, and Serene"

Overeating is often stress-driven. This recorded session will bring you into a calm and relaxed state, and then teach you how to re-create this wonderful state of relaxation in your everyday life. It will help you to become calmer and more focused by fostering balance, gratitude, and self-care.

Appendix C: FOOD EXCHANGES

Although this is by no means an exhaustive list, the foods listed below give you a general idea of the way food exchanges are categorized. There are many books, such as *Exchanges for All Occasions: Your Guide to Choosing Healthy Foods Anytime Anywhere,* by Marion J Franz, that can supply a more detailed list of food exchanges. Websites such as *www.mylifetime.com/shows/diettribe/your-food-exchange-list?page=0,0* will also give you a more comprehensive listing.

Carbohydrate Group

Starchy Carbohydrate List: One starch exchange has about 15 grams of carbohydrate and 3 grams of protein (80 calories).

- one slice of bread
- 1/2 hamburger or hotdog bun
- 3/4 cup of unsweetened cereal
- 1/3 cup pasta (cooked)
- 1 tortilla
- ½ pita bread (1 oz.)
- ¼ large bagel (1 oz.)
- ½ cup grits or oatmeal (cooked)
- 3 cups popcorn
- crackers (6 small saltines, 2 squares of graham crackers, 3 of most other crackers)
- 1 pancake or waffle (5-inch)

The vegetables included in the starch exchanges include:

- corn (1/2 cup or one ear)
- white potato, small (1/2 cup mashed)
- yam or sweet potato (1/2 cup)
- peas (1/2 cup)
- squash (1 cup)

- dried beans (1/2 cup)

Fruit List: 1 fruit exchange contains about 15 grams of carbohydrate (60 calories) and has essentially no fat or protein. Examples of one fruit exchange are:

- 1 small apple
- orange, pear, peach, or nectarine
- ½ banana
- ½ cup berries
- 1/3 of a small cantaloupe
- ¼ cup of watermelon
- 17 small grapes
- ½ grapefruit
- 2 tablespoons raisins
- 3 prunes

Vegetable List: With the exception of the vegetables listed above as starchy carbohydrates, ½ cup of cooked vegetables and one cup raw has about 5 grams of carbohydrate and 2 grams of protein (25 calories) and is considered 1 exchange. Below is a partial list of common vegetables:

- Artichoke
- Artichoke hearts
- Asparagus
- Bamboo shoots
- Beans: green, Italian, wax
- Broccoli
- Brussels sprouts
- Cabbage: bok choy, Chinese, green
- Carrots
- Cauliflower
- Celery
- Cucumber
- Eggplant
- Green onions or scallions

- Greens: collard, kale, mustard, turnip
- Jicama
- Leeks
- Mung bean sprouts
- Mushrooms
- Okra
- Onions
- Oriental radish or daikon
- Pea pods
- Peppers, all varieties
- Radishes
- Rutabaga
- Sauerkraut
- Spinach
- Sugar snap peas
- Summer squash
- Swiss chard
- Tomato: raw, canned, sauce, juice
- Turnips
- Vegetable juice cocktail
- Water chestnuts
- Zucchini

Protein Group

Proteins are divided into very lean proteins, lean proteins, medium-fat proteins, and high-fat proteins.

The **Very Lean** protein group includes foods that contain 7 grams of protein and 0 to 1 gram of fat (35 calories), for 1 exchange. Examples include:
- 1 ounce poultry (white meat, no skin)
- Fish fillet (flounder, sole, scrod, cod, etc.)
- Shellfish (clams, lobster, scallop, shrimp)
- 1 ounce tuna, canned in water

- 1 ounce fat-free cheese

The **Lean** protein group includes foods that contain 7 grams of protein and 3 grams of fat (55 calories), for 1 meat exchange. Examples include:

- 1 ounce poultry (dark meat, no skin)
- Salmon, swordfish, herring
- 1 ounce lean pork
- 1 ounce USDA Select or Choice grades of lean beef
- 1 ounce tuna, canned in oil, drained
- 1 ounce 4.5% fat cottage cheese

The **Medium-Fat** protein group includes foods that have 7 grams of protein and 5 grams of fat (75 calories). Examples include:

- 1 ounce beef (any prime cut), corned beef, ground beef
- 1 ounce pork chop
- ¼ cup ricotta cheese
- 1 ounce of low-fat cheese
- 1 egg
- 4 ounces tofu

The **High-Fat** group includes foods with 7 grams of protein and 8 grams of fat (100 calories). This group includes:

- 1 ounce pork sausage
- 1 ounce spare ribs
- 1 ounce fried fish
- 1 ounce regular cheese (American, Swiss etc.)
- 1 ounce lunch meat
- 1 ounce frankfurter or bratwurst

Fat Group

One fat exchange is equal to 5 grams of fat (45 calories). This group includes:

- ½ tablespoon nut butter—peanut, almond, cashew, macadamia, etc.
- 6 almonds
- 1 teaspoon oil (olive, peanut, canola)
- 1 teaspoon butter
- 1 strip of bacon
- 2 tablespoons of cream (half-and-half)
- 8 large black olives
- 1/8 avocado

Appendix D: RECOMMENDED RESOURCES

Books

NUTRITION

Bowden, Jonny. *Jonny Bowden's Shape Up!: The 8-week Program To Transform Your Body, Your Health, And Your Life.* Cambridge MA: Perseus Publishing, 2001.

DesMaisons, Kathleen. *Potatoes Not Prozac: How to Control Depression, Food Cravings and Weight Gain.* New York: Simon & Schuster, 2001.

Franz, Marion J. *Exchanges for All Occasions: Your Guide to Choosing Healthy Foods Anytime Anywhere.* St. Louis Park, MN: International Diabetes Center, 1997.

Gittleman, Ann Louise, M.S., C.N.S. *The Fat Flush Plan.* New York: McGraw Hill, 2002.

Hyman, Mark, M. D. *Ultra-Metabolism; The Simple Plan for Automatic Weight Loss.* New York: Atria Books, 2006.

Pollan, Michael. *In Defense of Food: An Eater's Manifesto.* New York: Penguin, 2009.

Ross, Julia. *The Diet Cure.* New York: Penguin, 2000.

Taubes, Gary. *Why We Get Fat: And What to Do About It.* Random House, 2010.

COOKBOOKS

Bowden, Jonny. *The 150 Healthiest Foods on the Earth; The Surprising, Unbiased Truth About What You Should Eat and Why.* Gloucester, MA: Fair Winds Press, 2007.

Carpender, Dana. *500 Low-Carb Recipes: 500 Recipes from Snacks to Dessert, That the Whole Family Will Love.* Fair Winds Press, 2002.

EMOTIONAL EATING

Roth, Geneen. *When You Eat at the Refrigerator, Pull Up a Chair: 50 Ways to Feel Thin, Gorgeous, and Happy (When You Feel Anything But).* New York: Hyperion, 1999.

--- - *Feeding the Hungry Heart: The Experience of Compulsive Eating.* New York: Penguin Books, 1982.

O'Malley, Mary. *The Gift of Our Compulsions: A Revolutionary Approach to Self-Acceptance and Healing.* New World Library, 2004.

EXERCISE

Bowden, Jonny. *Jonny Bowden's Shape Up! The 8-Week Program To Transform Your Body, Your Health, And Your Life.* Cambridge MA: Perseus Publishing, 2001.

Gerrish, Michael. *When Working Out Isn't Working Out: A Mind/Body Guide to Conquering Unidentified Fitness Obstacles.* New York: St. Martin's Griffin, 1999.

Neporent, Liz, Suzanne Schlosberg, and Shirley Archer. *Weight Training for Dummies.* Indianapolis, IN: Wiley Publishing, 2006.

EFT

Ball, Ron. *Freedom at Your Fingertips; Get Rapid Physical and Emotional Health With the Breakthrough System of Tapping.* Fredericksburg, VA: Inroads Publishing, 2006.

Carrington, Patricia, Ph.D. *EFT Choices Manual.* (ebook) *www.store.tappingcentral.com/choicesmethod.aspx*

Craig, Gary. *The EFT Manual (EFT: Emotional Freedom Techniques).* Fulton, CA: Energy Psychology Press, 2008.

--- *EFT for Weight Loss (EFT: Emotional Freedom Techniques).* Fulton, CA: Energy Psychology Press, 2010.

Feinstein, David, Donna Eden, and Gary Craig. *The Promise of Energy Psychology: Revolutionary Tools for Dramatic Personal Change.* New York: Jeremy P. Tarcher/The Penguin Group, 2005.

Hartmann, Sylvia. *Adventures in EFT: The Essential Field Guide to Emotional Freedom Techniques.* Charleston, SC: Booksurge, 2000.

Moore-Hafter, Betty. *Tapping Your Amazing Potential With EFT; Creative Ideas for Using Emotional Freedom Technique and Concepts from Hypnotherapy.* Burlington, VT: 2003. *www.creativeeft.com/eft-store_EFTManual.php*

MIND POWER

Hadley, Josie, and Carol Staudacher. *Hypnosis for Change.* New Age Books, 2002.

Hiatt, Marta, Ph.D. *Mind Magic; Techniques for Transforming Your Life.* New York: Llewellyn Publications, 2001.

Naparstek, Belleruth. *Staying Well with Guided Imagery.* New York: Grand Central Publishing, 1995.

Rossman, Martin L., M.D. *Guided Imagery for Self-Healing.* Novato, CA: HJ Kramer/New World Library, 2000.

Temes, Roberta, Ph.D. *The Complete Idiot's Guide to Hypnosis.* New York: Alpha Books, 2004.

MEDITATION AND YOGA

Brach, Tara, Ph.D. *Radical Acceptance: Embracing Your Life with the Heart of a Buddha.* New York: Bantam Books, 2003.

Cope, Stephen. *Yoga and the Quest for the True Self.* New York: Bantam, 2000.

--- *The Wisdom of Yoga: A Seeker's Guide to Extraordinary Living.* New York: Bantam, 2007.

Farhi, Donna. *Yoga Mind, Body & Spirit: A Return to Wholeness.* New York: Holt Paperbacks, 2000.

Goldstein, Joseph. *Insight Meditation: The Practice of Freedom.* Boston: Shambhala, 2003.

Kornfield, Jack. *Meditation for Beginners.* Louisville, CO: Sounds True, Incorporated, 2008.

Lasater, Judith Hanson P.T., Ph.D. *Living Your Yoga: Finding the Spiritual in Everyday Life.* Berkeley, CA: Rodmell Press, 1999.

Levine, Stephen. *Guided Meditations, Explorations and Healings.* New York: Anchor, 1991.

Salzberg, Susan. *Lovingkindness: The Revolutionary Art of Happiness.* Boston, MA: Shambhala, 2008.

STRESS MANAGEMENT

Charlesworth, Edward A. and Ronald G. Nathan. *Stress Management: A Comprehensive Guide to Wellness.* New York: Ballantine Books, 2004.

Davis, Martha, Ph.D., Elizabeth R. Eshelman, M.S.W., and Matthew McKay, Ph.D. *The Relaxation and Stress Reduction Workbook.* New York: New Harbinger Publications, 1994.

Domar, Alice, Ph.D. *Healing Mind, Healthy Woman: Using the Mind-Body Connection to Manage Stress and Take Control of Your Life.* New York: Henry Holt and Company, 1996.

Websites

NUTRITION

Dr. Jonny Bowden's Blog
Jonny Bowden is one of my very favorite nutritionists. He is extremely knowledgeable, yet down-to-earth, and can explain complicated scientific data in clear terms that everyone can comprehend.
www.jonnybowdenblog.com

Jimmy Moore's Livin' La Vida Low Carb Blog and Podcast
Low-carb diets are low-glycemic diets, so even if you don't follow a diet like Atkins or South Beach, you'll still find the information on these blog and podcast sites extremely valuable and entertaining.
www.livinlavidalowcarb.com/blog
www.thelivinlowcarbshow.com/shownotes

About.com: Low-Carb Diets

This is Laura Dolson's Low Carb site. It is another very informative site, with great nutrition information and recipe ideas.
www.lowcarbdiets.about.com

Slow Food Movement

Slow Food is a non-profit, eco-gastronomic, member-supported organization that was founded in 1989 to counteract fast food and fast life, the disappearance of local food traditions, and people's dwindling interest in the food they eat, where it comes from, how it tastes and how our food choices affect the rest of the world. To do that, Slow Food links pleasure and responsibility, and makes them inseparable.
www.slowfood.com

Glycemic Load

This is the definitive table for both the glycemic index and the glycemic load.
www.mendosa.com/gilists.htm

Food Exchanges

Here is a comprehensive Food Exchange List. Remember that this list was created by the American Diabetic and the American Dietetic Associations. Although I make use of their lists, I do not recommend the same percentage of food from each group, nor do I advocate their low-fat, high-carbohydrate approach to meal planning.
www.perinatology.com/Nutrition/EXCHANGE%20LIST.pdf

EXERCISE

Exercise Is Medicine

This organization is teaching and motivating the medical field to educate their patients about exercise in an effort to "make physi-

cal activity and exercise a standard part of a disease prevention and treatment medical paradigm in the United States."
www.ExerciseIsMedicine.org
This is the very informative "Keys to Exercise Video" page.
www.exerciseismedicine.org/keys.htm

American Council on Exercise (ACE)

Although the ACE site is geared primarily toward exercise professionals, the page below provides lots of information on exercise, including research, workouts, and an exercise library.
www.acefitness.org/getfit/default.aspx
And if you're looking for an ACE-certified personal trainer, you can search for one in your area from this page:
www.acefitness.org/findanacepro/default.aspx

American College of Sports Medicine (ACSM)

This is another site for fitness professionals. The following link is geared toward educating the public about how to exercise safely and effectively:
www.acsm.org/AM/Template.cfm?Section=General_Public

And if you're looking for an ACESM-certified personal trainer (like me!), you can search for one in your area from this page:
www.forms.acsm.org/_frm/crt/online_locator.asp

Fitness Wholesale

Fitness Wholesale offers a wide variety of fitness equipment, books and videos at reasonable prices.
www.fwonline.com

Perform Better

Another excellent site for fitness equipment, books and videos, with an emphasis on sport-specific and functional training
http://www.performbetter.com

Collage Video
This is a really great website for exercise videos. Every video is examined by an ACE-certified instructor and categorized according to type, length, level of difficulty, and overall quality
www.collagevideo.com

EFT and HYPNOSIS

EFT Universe
EFT Universe is the website to which EFT founder Gary Craig entrusted the archives of EFT when he retired. It is owned and maintained by Energy Psychology Press, and provides a wealth of information and resources for both experienced and new EFT users.

On this site, you can sample cases written by everyday people, as well as therapists, doctors, nurses, and mental health professionals who have had success with EFT. You can also sign up to receive the invaluable EFT Insights Newsletter, hosted by David MacKay.
www.eftuniverse.com

EFTfree.net
In an effort to continue Gary's generous efforts to provide information about EFT at little or no cost, three talented EFT practitioners put together this site as an educational web resource, featuring articles from professional practitioners and EFT explorers from all over the world.
www.eftfree.net

EFT Founding Masters
The EFT Founding Masters are certified EFT practitioners, therapists, trainers and coaches dedicated to inspiring the mastery, understanding and creative expansion of EFT worldwide. This

site offers information about creative and often unique applications of EFT.
www.eftmastersworldwide.com

Rising Sun Healing

This is Betty Moore-Hafter's website. Betty is one of my favorite hypnotherapists and EFT practitioners, and does a superb job of synthesizing these two skills in her work. *www.creativeeft.com*

Energy Therapies Associates

This is the site of two skilled and insightful therapist and EFT practitioners in Arlington, MA. Not only are they fantastic therapists, they also offer live EFT trainings in the Boston area.
www.energytherapyassociates.com

MEDITATION, MINDFULNESS, and YOGA

Learning Meditation

This site contains a series of fairly short, guided meditations. A good place to begin if you're new to this practice.
www.learningmeditation.com

How to Meditate

This site offers practical information about Buddhist meditation that is clear, simple and easy to understand. Its goal is to "make Buddhist meditation more accessible to busy people."
www.how-to-meditate.org

The Center for Mindful Eating

This is a forum for people interested in developing, deepening, and understanding the value and importance of mindful eating.
http://www.tcme.org

Yoga Journal

This site is filled to the brim with all things yoga. It contains great articles and videos, and describes itself as "your online retreat for yoga poses, classes, meditation, and life—on and off the mat." *www.yogajournal.com*

Sounds True

Sounds True is an independent multimedia publishing company that embraces the world's major spiritual traditions, as well as the arts and humanities, embodied by the leading authors, teachers, and visionary artists of our time. It sells a wide variety of books, video and audio products to "inspire, support, and serve continuous spiritual awakening and its expression in the world." *www.soundstrue.com*

STRESS MANAGEMENT

Inner Health Studio

This comprehensive site provides a wide variety of free relaxation scripts, audio and video downloads, and self-help techniques for managing stress. *www.innerhealthstudio.com*

About.com: Stress Management

This is Elizabeth Scott's very informative stress-management site. It contains information about causes and effects of stress and a comprehensive resource of stress-management techniques. *www.stress.about.com/bio/Elizabeth-Scott-M-S-17577.htm*

Bibliography

Aerobics and Fitness Association of America. *Fitness Theory and Practice*. Sherman Oaks, CA: Aerobics & Fitness Assn of Amer, 1997.

American College Sports Medicine. *ACSM's Health-Related Physical Fitness Assessment Manual*. Philadelphia: Lippincott Williams & Wilkins, 2009.

--- *ACSM's Guidelines for Exercise Testing and Prescription*. Philadelphia: Lippincott Williams & Wilkins, 2009.

--- *ACSM's Resources for the Personal Trainer*. Philadelphia: Lippincott Williams & Wilkins, 2009.

Agatston, Arthur, M.D. *The South Beach Diet: The Delicious, Doctor-Designed, Foolproof Plan for Fast and Healthy Weight Loss*. New York: Rodale, Inc., 2003.

Alter, Judy. *Stretch and Strengthen*. Boston, MA: Mariner Books, 1992.

Anderson, Bob. *Stretching*. Bolinas, CA: Shelter Publications, 2000.

Atkins, Robert, M.D. *Dr. Atkins' New Diet Revolution*. New York: Bantam Books, 1992.

Ball, Ron. *Freedom at Your Fingertips; Get Rapid Physical and Emotional Health With the Breakthrough System of Tapping*. Fredericksburg, VA: Inroads Publishing, 2006.

Banyan, Calvin D. and Gerald F. Klein. *Hypnosis and Hypnotherapy Basic to Advanced Techniques for the Professional*. Scroggins, TX: Abbot Publishing House, 2001.

Bowden, Jonny, C.N.S. *Living the Low Carb Life: Controlled Carbohydrate Eating for Long-Term Weight Loss.* New York: Sterling, 2004.

--- *Jonny Bowden's Shape Up! The 8-Week Program To Transform Your Body, Your Health, And Your Life.* Cambridge MA: Perseus Publishing, 2001.

--- *The 150 Healthiest Foods on the Earth; The Surprising, Unbiased Truth About What You Should Eat and Why.* Gloucester, MA: Fair Winds Press, 2007.

Brach, Tara, Ph.D. *Radical Acceptance: Embracing Your Life with the Heart of a Buddha.* New York: Bantam Books, 2003.

Brill, Peggy, P.T. and Gerald Secor Couzens. *The Core Program: Fifteen Minutes a Day That Can Change Your Life.* New York: Bantam, 2003.

Broadhurst, Leigh, Ph.D. *Diabetes: Prevention and Cure.* New York: Kensington Books, 1999.

Carrington, Patricia, Ph.D. *EFT Choices Manual.* (ebook) *www.store.tappingcentral.com/choicesmethod.aspx*

Challem, Jack, Burton Berkson, and Melissa D. Smith. *Syndrome X: The Complete Nutritional Program to Prevent and Reverse Insulin Resistance.* Hoboken, NJ: Wiley, 2001.

Challem, Jack. *The Inflammation Syndrome: Your Nutrition Plan for Great Health, Weight Loss, and Pain-Free Living.* Wiley, 2010.

Charlesworth, Edward A. and Ronald G. Nathan. *Stress Management: A Comprehensive Guide to Wellness.* New York: Ballantine Books, 2004.

Clark, Nancy, M.S., R.D. *Nancy Clark's Sports Nutrition Guidebook.* Champaign, IL: Human Kinetics, 1990.

Cope, Stephen. *Yoga and the Quest for the True Self.* New York: Bantam, 2000.

--- *The Wisdom of Yoga: A Seeker's Guide to Extraordinary Living.* New York: Bantam, 2007.

Crayhon, Robert. *Nutrition Made Simple.* New York: M. Evans and Company, Inc., 1994.

Craig, Gary. *The EFT Manual (EFT: Emotional Freedom Techniques).* Fulton, CA: Energy Psychology Press, 2008.

--- EFT for Weight Loss (EFT: Emotional Freedom Techniques). Fulton, CA: Energy Psychology Press, 2010.

Dass, Ram. *Journey of Awakening: A Meditator's Guidebook.* New York: Bantam, 1990.

Davich, Victor N. *The Best Guide to Meditation.* Riverside, CA: Renaissance Books, 1998.
Davis, Martha, Ph.D., Elizabeth R. Eshelman, M.S.W., and Matthew McKay, Ph.D. *The Relaxation and Stress Reduction Workbook.* New York: New Harbinger Publications, 1994.

Desikacher, T.K.V. *The Heart of Yoga: Developing a Personal Practice.* Rochester, VT: Inner Traditions, 1999

DesMaisons, Kathleen, Ph.D. *Your Last Diet.* New York: Ballantine Publishing Group, 2001.

--- *Potatoes Not Prozac: How to Control Depression, Food Cravings and Weight Gain.* New York: Simon & Schuster, 2001.

Domar, Alice, Ph.D. *Healing Mind, Healthy Woman: Using the Mind-Body Connection to Manage Stress and Take Control of Your Life.* New York: Henry Holt and Company, 1996.

Domar, Alice and Henry Dreher. *Self-Nurture: Learning to Care for Yourself As Effectively As You Care for Everyone Else.* New York: Penguin, 2001.

Eades, Michael, M.D. and Mary Eades, M.D. *Protein Power.* New York: Bantam Books, 1999.

--- *The Protein Power Life Plan.* New York: Warner Books, 2000.

Elias, Jack. *Finding True Magic: Transpersonal Hypnosis and Hypnotherapy/NLP.* Seattle, WA: Five Wisdoms Press, 2005.

Feinstein, David, Donna Eden, and Gary Craig. *The Promise of Energy Psychology: Revolutionary Tools for Dramatic Personal Change.* New York: Jeremy P. Tarcher/The Penguin Group, 2005.

Farhi, Donna. *Yoga Mind, Body & Spirit: A Return to Wholeness.* New York: Holt Paperbacks, 2000.

Fletcher, Ann M. *Thin for Life.* Vermont: Chapters Publishing, Ltd., 1994.

Franz, Marion J. *Exchanges for All Occasions: Your Guide to Choosing Healthy Foods Anytime Anywhere.* St. Louis Park, MN: International Diabetes Center, 1997.

Fraser, Laura. *Losing It: America's Obsession with Weight and the Industry That Feeds On It.* New York: Penguin Group, 1997.

Gallo, Fred P. and Harry Vincenzi. *Energy Tapping.* Oakland, CA: New Harbinger Publications, 2000.

Gerrish, Michael. *When Working Out Isn't Working Out: A Mind/Body Guide to Conquering Unidentified Fitness Obstacles.* New York: St. Martin's Griffin, 1999.

Ginsburg, Lynn and Mary Taylor. *What Are You Hungry For?* New York: St. Martin's Press, 2002.

Gittleman, Ann Louise, M.S., C.N.S. *The Fat Flush Plan.* New York: McGraw Hill, 2002.

--- *Guide to the 40/30/30 Phenomenon.* New York: Contemporary Books, 2002.

Griffin, Julie. *Facilitating Wellness: Inside the Miracle of Hypnosis.* Pelham, NH: TWT Publishing, 1997.

--- *Recipes for Weight Loss.* Pelham, NH: TWT Publishing, 1997.

Goldstein, Joseph. *Insight Meditation: The Practice of Freedom.* Boston, MA: Shambhala, 2003.

Hadley, Josie, and Carol Staudacher. *Hypnosis for Change.* New Age Books, 2002.

Hahn, Frederick, Mary Eades, and Michael R. Eades. *The Slow Burn Fitness Revolution: The Slow Motion Exercise That Will Change Your Body in 30 Minutes a Week.* New York: Random House, 2002.

Hartmann, Sylvia. *Adventures in EFT: The Essential Field Guide to Emotional Freedom Techniques.* Charleston, SC: Booksurge, 2000.

Hass, Elson, M.D. *The False Fat Diet: The Revolutionary 21-Day Program for Losing the Weight You Think Is Fat.* New York: Ballantine Books, 2001.

Heller, Richard, M.D. and Rachel Heller, M.D. *The Carbohydrate Addict's Diet: The Lifelong Solution to Yo-Yo Dieting.* New York: Penguin Books, 1995.

Hiatt, Marta, Ph.D. *Mind Magic; Techniques for Transforming Your Life.* New York: Llewellyn Publications, 2001.

Hirschmann, Jane R., and Carol H. Munter. *When Women Stop Hating Their Bodies; Freeing Yourself from Food and Weight Obsession.* New York: Ballantine Books, 1997.

Hogan, Kevin. *The New Hypnotherapy Handbook: Hypnosis and Mind/Body Healing.* Eagan, MN: Network 3000, May 2001.

Hyman, Mark, M. D. *Ultra-Metabolism; The Simple Plan for Automatic Weight Loss.* New York: Atria Books, 2006.

Kabatznick, Ronna, Ph.D. *The Zen of Eating.* New York: Berkley Publishing, 1998.

Kessler, David. *The End of Overeating: Taking Control of the Insatiable American Appetite.* Rodale Books, 2010.

Kraftsow, Gary. *Yoga for Wellness: Healing with the Timeless Teachings of Viniyoga.* New York: Penguin, 1999.

--- *Yoga for Transformation: Ancient Teachings and Practices for Healing the Body, Mind, and Heart.* New York: Penguin, 2002.

Kornfield, Jack. *Meditation for Beginners.* Louisville, CO: Sounds True, Incorporated, 2008.

Lasater, Judith Hanson P.T., Ph.D. *Living Your Yoga: Finding the Spiritual in Everyday Life.* Berkeley, CA: Rodmell Press, 1999.

--- *Relax and Renew: Restful Yoga for Stressful Times*. Berkeley, CA: Rodmell Press, 1995.

Levey, Joel, and Michelle Levey. *Living in Balance: A Dynamic Approach for Creating Harmony & Wholeness in a Chaotic World*. Newburyport, MA: Conari Press, 1998.

Levine, Stephen. *Guided Meditations, Explorations and Healings*. New York: Anchor, 1991.

Look, Carol. *How to Lose Weight with Energy Therapy*. New York: 2001. (available from Carol's website)

McCullough, Fran. *The Good Fat Cookbook*. New York: Scribner, 2003.

Manning, George, Kent Curtis, and Steve McMillen. *Stress: Living and Working in a Changing World*. Duluth, MN: Whole Person Associates, 1998.

Mellin, Laurel, M.A., R.D. *The Solution: Six Winning Ways to Permanent Weight Loss*. New York: Harper Collins Publishing, 1997.

Mercola, Joseph, M.D. *The No-Grain Diet: Conquer Carbohydrate Addiction and Stay Slim for Life*. New York: Dutton, 2003.

--- *Dr. Mercola's Total Health Cookbook and Program*. Hoffman Estates, IL: Mercola.com, 2003-2004.

Moore-Hafter, Betty. *Tapping Your Amazing Potential With EFT; Creative Ideas for Using Emotional Freedom Technique and Concepts from Hypnotherapy*. Burlington, VT: 2003.

Naparstek, Belleruth. *Staying Well with Guided Imagery*. New York: Grand Central Publishing, 1995.

Neporent, Liz, Suzanne Schlosberg, and Shirley Archer. *Weight Training for Dummies*. Indianapolis, IN: Wiley Publishing, 2006.

O'Connor, Richard, Ph.D. *Undoing Perpetual Stress; The Missing Connection Between Depression, Anxiety, and 21st Century Illness*. New York: Berkeley Books, 2005.

O'Malley, Mary. *The Gift of Our Compulsions; A Revolutionary Approach to Self-Acceptance and Healing*. Novato, CA: New World Library, 2004.

Ornish, Dean, M.D. *Eat More, Weigh Less*. New York: Harper Perennial, 1994.

Peak, Pamela, M.D., M.P.H. *Fight Fat After Forty*. New York: Penguin Group, 2000.

Pollan, Michael. *In Defense of Food: An Eater's Manifesto*. New York: Penguin, 2009.

Reaven, Gerald, M.D. *Syndrome X*. New York: Simon and Schuster, 2000.

Richards, Byron J., and Mary Guignon Richards. *Mastering Leptin: Your Guide to Permanent Weight Loss and Optimum Health*. Minneapolis: Wellness Resources Books, 2009.

Ross, Julia. *The Diet Cure*. New York: Penguin, 2000.

Rossman, Martin L., M.D. *Guided Imagery for Self-Healing*. Novato, CA: HJ Kramer/New World Library, 2000.

Roth, Geneen. *When Food Is Love: Exploring the Relationship Between Eating and Intimacy*. New York: Dutton Books, 1991.

--- *Feeding the Hungry Heart: The Experience of Compulsive Eating.*
New York: Penguin Books, 1982.

--- *When You Eat at the Refrigerator, Pull Up a Chair.* New York:
Hyperion, 1993.

--- *Breaking Free from Compulsive Eating.* New York: Plume, 1993.

Salzberg ,Susan. *Lovingkindness: The Revolutionary Art of Happiness.*
Boston, MA: Shambhala, 2008.

Sears, Barry, M.D. *Enter the Zone: A Dietary Road Map.* New York:
Harper Collins, 1995.

Shomon, Mary J. *The Thyroid Diet: Manage Your Metabolism for Lasting Weight Loss.* New York: Harper Paperbacks, 2004.

--- *The Soy Zone.* New York: Penguin Books, 2000.

Somer, Elizabeth, M.A., R.D. *Food & Mood: The Complete Guide to
Eating Well and Feeling Your Best.* New York: Holt Paperbacks,
1999.

Talbott, Shawn, Ph.D. *The Cortisol Connection; The Breakthrough Program to Control Stress and Lose Weight.* Berkeley, CA: Group West,
2004.

Taubes, Gary. *Good Calories, Bad Calories: Fats, Carbs, and the Contro-
versial Science of Diet and Health.* New York: Anchor, 2008.

--- *Why We Get Fat: And What to Do About It.* Random House,
2010.

Temes, Roberta, Ph.D. *The Complete Idiot's Guide to Hypnosis.* New
York: Alpha Books, 2004.

Tribole, Evelyn, M.S., R.D., and Elyse Resch, M.S., R.D. *Intuitive Eating: A Recovery Book for the Chronic Dieter.* New York: St. Martin's Press, 1995.

Verstegen, Mark and Pete Williams. *The Core Performance: The Revolutionary Workout Program to Transform Your Body & Your Life.* Red Oak, IA: Rodale Books, 2005.

Weiss, Andrew. *Beginning Mindfulness: Learning the Way of Awareness.* Novato, CA: New World Library, 2004.

Willet, Walter, M.D. *Eat, Drink and Be Healthy: The Harvard Medical School Guide to Healthy Eating.* New York: Simon and Schuster, 2001.

Young, Lisa, Ph.D. *The Portion Teller: Smartsize Your Way to Permanent Weight Loss.* New York: Morgan Road Books, 2005.

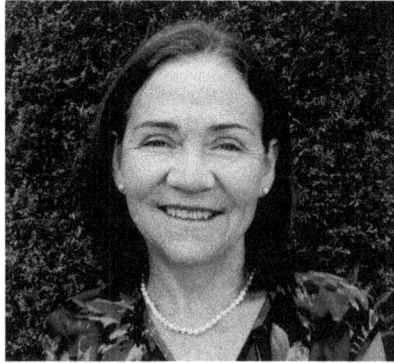

About the Author

Terry L Currier is a personal trainer, hypnotherapist, Emotional Freedom Techniques (EFT) practitioner, and yoga teacher. She has combined her extensive knowledge and experience in the fitness industry with her training in alternative therapies to create a powerful, effective weight loss program that addresses both the physical and emotional aspects of losing weight.

Website: _www.tlcweightloss.net_
Email: _terry@tlcweightloss.net_

www.ingramcontent.com/pod-product-compliance
Lightning Source LLC
Chambersburg PA
CBHW062215270326
41930CB00009B/1744